SOS FOR YOUR HORMONAL HOT MESS

Your Ultimate Rescue Guide for PMS, PCOS and Menopause

KATHY RYAN AND
DARPAN AHLUWALIA

LUCKY BOOK PUBLISHING

Published by Lucky Book Publishing: www.luckybookpublishing.com

To request permissions, contact the publisher at hello@luckybookpublishing.com.

Paperback ISBN: 978-1-998287-37-6
Hardcover ISBN: 978-1-998287-36-9
E-book ISBN: 978-1-998287-38-3

1st edition, October 2024.

MY GIFT TO YOU

I am so glad you're here!

As my Gift to you, get FREE Access to the Audiobook of SOS for Your Hormonal Hot Mess by scanning the QR Code below or visiting

HormoneBook.com/book

PRAISE FOR SOS FOR YOUR HORMONAL HOT MESS

"This book is an invaluable resource for women seeking to reclaim their health and well-being. Written in an accessible style, it serves as a proactive guide that empowers readers to take control of their bodies.It offers women a unique opportunity to understand and reclaim their health by providing clear insights into the complexities of our bodies.

As a postmenopausal woman, I recognize that one of the significant challenges many women face are accessing reliable, practical information regarding hormonal imbalances. This book addresses that gap, equipping readers with a wealth of quality information grounded in both natural therapies and scientific expertise. It puts you in the driver's seat, enabling you to navigate your health journey with confidence."

- Shelley A Mudock, Best-Selling Author, HEALTHY & FIT FOR LIFE-THE STARTER KIT FOR WOMEN OVER 50

"It didn't even get to the first chapter before I was hooked. It was my life described here. I just wish I had this information when I was 15. This is an amazing book, so much information that will make your life better. Now at 50 I finally have a solution. I have read and heard about Darpan before but now I will be make an appointment with her. A must read for every woman."

- Nadee Fernando-O'Driscoll, Author, Labyrinth of Dreams

"Finally, a comprehensive guide for women struggling with hormonal imbalances! Kathy and Darpan sheds light on the often-misunderstood connection between hormones and mood, energy, and overall well-being. A must-read for those looking to reclaim balance naturally."

- Manali Haridas, CEO, Zen for You & Author of " You Got This Mom" Handbook

"SOS For Your Hormone Hot Mess is the ultimate guide for navigating PMS, PCOS, and menopause. Darpan and Kathy reveal the critical role of hormones and offer natural solutions your doctor may not tell you. This book is empowering and life-changing."

- Cristie Vito, Keynote Speaker and Author - Bless the Meds

"From mood swings to menopausal weight gain, SOS For Your Hormone Hot Mess breaks down complex hormonal issues with clarity and compassion. The natural solutions offered are practical and effective—this is a guide every woman needs."

- Rosy, the Mortgageless Mentor, Author, Don't Have Sex Nine Months Before Christmas and other Practical Financial Tips

"Darpan and Kathy's book provides a refreshing take on hormone health, blending science with the energetic wisdom of the feminine cycle. SOS For Your Hormone Hot Mess is both educational and empowering—a must-have resource for every woman seeking balance."

- Sarah Boyd, Holistic Lifestyle Coach and Co-Founder of @thesocialwellnesscollective

"Finally, a book that dives deep into hormone health with empathy and expertise! SOS For Your Hormone Hot Mess is packed with invaluable tips on balancing hormones naturally, from thyroid support to adrenal health—this guide is a true lifesaver."

- Fran Garton, Pain Reduction Coach, Fibromyalgia Warrior and Body-Positive Trainer

"Practical, insightful, and easy to follow, SOS For Your Hormone Hot Mess offers a fresh perspective on hormone balance. Darpan and Kathy's advice on nutrition, supplements, and holistic approaches will help any woman struggling with hormone-related symptoms."

- Richa Rehan, Physiotherapist, Best-selling Author, Things Every Girl Should Know About Her Body: A Girl's Guide to Periods, Growing Up and Loving Your Body

"SOS For Your Hormone Hot Mess is a brilliant resource for understanding the underlying causes of hormone imbalances. Darpan and Kathy offer clear, actionable solutions for everything from PMS to menopause—an essential read for every woman!"

- Teri Kingston, TedX Speaker Coach, Best-selling Author, Get Ready for TED When TED is Ready for you!: Your Step-By-Step Guide to Getting Accepted so You Can Spread Your Idea around the World

"Darpan and Kathy's compassionate approach to hormone health is refreshing and timely. SOS For Your Hormone Hot Mess gives you the tools you need to decode your hormone symptoms and reclaim your energy and vitality. Highly recommended for every stage of womanhood."

> **- *Ellie Laliberté, Best-Selling Author, Letters From You to You: Awaken Your Power Through Conversations With Your Higher Self***

"This book does an amazing job of simplifying the complex world of hormones. It provides practical and effective steps you can easily implement! A must read for anyone who wants to take back control of their health."

> **- *Dr. Jonathan Beatty ND, Clinician, Instructor, NHP formulator***

Wonder Women, Wonder No More!

Everything you need to know about your hormones and how they affect you is captured in this gem of a book authored by Kathy & Darpan . Finally, women can gain the knowledge and understanding of our bodies, our hormones, our mood swings, our thyroid health—everything that connects us to living well is in this book.

When I was 22, I underwent a tubal ligation—a surgical procedure commonly referred to as "getting your tubes tied." Back then, no one understood why I couldn't carry our two children beyond seven months, why I was sick every day during that time, or why I needed a cesarean section. Today, we know it was a result of estrogen dominance. Fifty years ago, such awareness was unheard of.

As I approach my 70th year, I now understand the "whys." This book is going into the hands of my four granddaughters—to empower them with knowledge we didn't have. It includes everything from how diet impacts hormones to the best supplements to take.

You'll wonder no more, you superwomen! This book is truly empowering and life-changing."

- Lilly White, Archetype Consultant, Soul Coach, Author, creator of Power Up Your Life Events, Breakfast with Soul, Bali Spiritual guide

"This is the book every woman needs on her nightstand. Honest, empowering, and filled with expert guidance, it takes the mystery out of hormones and gives you the roadmap to reclaim your body and mind."

- Jennifer Agugliaro, Founder of FuDogGroup

ACKNOWLEDGMENTS

Many thanks to our mentors, guides, and clients who have both taught and shaped our approach to helping women understand and navigate their own hormonal health.

There is still much work to be done to empower women and girls to recognize the influence of their hormones on their physical and mental health, mood, and vitality. We are grateful to all the doctors, and other health providers who are offering women more choice when it comes to optimizing their hormonal health.

We extend heartfelt thanks to our respective families and our publishers for their unwavering support as we completed this book.

"When hormones are put back in balance, a woman or man resumes their life of feeling good and having days filled with quality."

~Suzanne Summers

INTRODUCTION: OUR STORIES ARE EVERY WOMAN'S STORY

Kathy's Story

The story I'm going to tell you is not unique.

It's a story I've heard a thousand times from women from all walks of life. It's a common story that tells me unequivocally something needs to change about the way we talk about and manage women's health and hormones.

The general lack of knowledge girls and women have about their bodies and the interplay between their hormones and their health is not ok. As a collective, we have placed our health into the hands of our modern medical system and have been taught to trust medical professionals and modern science above all else.

This is not a commentary about the medical professionals themselves—most who care deeply for their patients—but of a system that prioritizes "experts" and pharmaceuticals over our own innate wisdom and the natural cycles that have been in place since the dawn of humanity.

When the only options women are given to correct

their hormone imbalances involve artificially suppressing their cycles or removal of the offending organs—we have missed the mark. We need to do better.

I wrote this book to let you know:

You have options.

You're not crazy, lazy, mean or sick.

Your seemingly random symptoms are real and related.

And most importantly—you are not alone.

I was 12 when my menstrual cycle first started, and from day one there were issues. I didn't know it at the time because, apart from some whispers among my friends about what was normal and what wasn't, I didn't have any information at my disposal.

My cycle was 21 days long, and I had my period for a full week. This meant I had 14 days without a period, followed by seven days with a period. My periods were especially heavy, but I had no reference point and didn't know this until many years later.

Another thing I didn't know at the time was that if a girl was experiencing symptoms such as PMS, cramping, heavy bleeding or too frequent cycles—those symptoms were signs that something was wrong.

When something is wrong at 12 or 13 years old, it doesn't suddenly, magically get better the older a girl/woman gets. What starts off as heavy, too frequent periods or PMS can gradually turn into things like Polycystic Ovarian Syndrome, fibroids, endometriosis, difficulty getting pregnant, a difficult pregnancy or postpartum, hellish perimenopausal symptoms, mental health issues, autoimmune diagnosis, and even cancer.

When I work with women in their 40s and 50s who are experiencing extreme menopausal symptoms such as raging hot flashes, night sweats, insomnia, irritability, depression, and more—these things don't just come out of the blue. There is always a history of hormonal issues.

When I finally went to my doctor to discuss my concerns about my cycles, fatigue, IBS, facial hair, acne, and depression, I was told that I could go on the pill and that would solve all my problems. I opted not to, as even as a teen I had a resistance to medication and I didn't want what I called an "artificial" cycle.

Over the years I dealt with increasingly erratic cycles, high prolactin levels (with no discernible cause), low ferritin (iron stores), depression, and extreme fatigue, until at the age of 24 I started getting hot flashes. I laughed about this with my friends, like a big joke that I was "going through menopause," but little did I know that's exactly what was happening.

My cycles were worse than they had ever been. Sometimes I would bleed for 30+ days and then stop for five days and then bleed another eight days. I was away at school at the time in another province so I didn't go to a doctor. It was awful. I was exhausted and honestly broke just from having to buy so many period supplies on a student income. When I returned home after my final semester, I finally agreed to go on the pill, as my doctor told me if this didn't stop I would be looking at an early hysterectomy.

So I went on the pill because this was the only option given to me. But nobody told me how the pill might impact my moods or that the pill depleted important nutrients that I needed to be healthy and happy. Sure, I was thankful that I wasn't bleeding 30 days at a time anymore, but I was constantly irritated, always on edge, always fighting to be in a good mood.

I was newly engaged and planning a wedding. This should have been a really amazing time, but everything stressed me out. Everything bothered me. I had no patience and desperately wanted to be happy, kind, patient, and fun. I had no idea this personality change had anything to do with being on the pill.

I stayed on the pill for less than a year. I was already worried about my ability to have children, and I wanted to do everything I could to support that eventual goal. As soon as I came off it, the constant irritation left and I felt more like myself again. My issues with my cycles came back with a vengeance—but thankfully a surprise pregnancy put a halt to everything.

Getting pregnant wasn't something I wanted to do "yet," but looking back it was the best possible thing that could have happened. When I was pregnant I felt incredible. I was calm, happy and even blissful. Nothing bothered me. I was six months pregnant when my husband left for three months to go to police college. The date he started police college was September 11, 2001. We didn't know what the future held or how the world would change, but we were thrilled to welcome our daughter in January 2002.

Postpartum was rough. I was a new mother in a new city with my husband working night shifts and overtime. After a blissful pregnancy, I had a traumatic birth. Everybody talked about "postpartum depression," but it seemed like everyone I knew had this and I refused to be lumped in with everyone else—and by this point I had become very antimedication. So I just dealt with the ongoing fatigue and chalked the low mood and crying jags up to the fact that I was "adjusting" to this new life, in a new city, as a new mother, with a husband in a high-stress job.

I nursed my daughter for two years, and when she was nine months old, my cycles came back. I was worried about what their return would be like, but they were the lightest and least "intrusive" to my life they had ever been. Unexpectedly, the very month I weaned her, my cycles stopped. I thought I was pregnant again, but a blood test showed my hormones were at postmenopausal levels. After further testing, it was determined that I had a genetic condition that put me into premature ovarian failure.

Going through perimenopause in my twenties was not fun. The hot flashes and night sweats were a level 10 out of 10. I was back to feeling exhausted and irritated. I had brain fog, crying jags, and depression and lost my joy for everything. I had additional scary symptoms like extreme muscle weakness that would randomly come and go. I was tested for MS and other neurological disorders, but everything came back negative. My marriage that I was sure could withstand anything thrown at it quickly disintegrated into divorce, and I was passed from doctor to doctor who tried all manner of hormone replacement to deal with my most pressing symptoms and address their singular-focused mandate to "protect my bones."

The problem was, I could not tolerate progestins which I was told were a must in my HRT (hormone replacement therapy) protocol. Progestins are a synthetic form of progesterone that I was told was "the same" as my own progesterone, but I learned that was definitely not the case.

Progestins were in the birth control pill I had used years earlier that had changed my personality and made me moody and irritated. But now, the symptoms were magnified to an extreme. After only one week on the first round of HRT they tried me on, I wanted to die. Only I knew I didn't really want to die. I knew something was wrong. I felt completely unhinged. I knew I was reacting to the HRT.

My doctor agreed, and after being off it for a week, I was back to normal. This process repeated itself three more times as they tried me on different combinations and dosages—all with the same disastrous results. I was then referred to the women's health clinic at our local hospital and was told the next step was to try a mirena IUD because the progestin level was much lower and more localized.

I told the doctor treating me that my reaction to progestins was extreme. It was dangerous. I asked him how long would I have to wait to get in to see him to get the IUD removed if I couldn't tolerate it. His response shocked me. He said I had to wait three months for my body to "get used to" the hormones and that he wouldn't take it out until after I tried it for three months.

I told him that I couldn't do that. I explained, again, that this was not simply a case of being irritated, or in a low mood. This was life and death. He became frustrated with me and told me it was three months or nothing. I chose nothing. He dismissed me as a patient and told me I was on my own.

It was at that point that I went on a mission to learn everything I could about hormones—not just to heal myself but to understand all the options that existed that we were not being told about. Many options that our doctors don't know anything about. Options that exist beyond medication or surgeries. Options that changed my life and that have changed the lives of thousands of other women for the better.

Darpan's Story

Since the age of 15, prioritizing my health and harnessing the power of vitamins, herbs, and proper food have been at the center of my life. Even as a teenager, I was the go-to person for advice on wellness—helping friends, family, and clients because I was so passionate and knowledgeable about the power of natural remedies.

A big part of my motivation was watching the women in my family and inner circle struggle with weight, hormonal imbalances, and other health issues. My mother had a partial hysterectomy in her late 40s, and her own mother, my grandmother, had also faced the same fate. My sister suffered for years with excruciating pain, fevers, and heavy bleeding during her cycles, often missing school for three to four days every month. We didn't know it at the time, but she was eventually diagnosed with PCOS. I learned in my studies about how hormonal issues were often genetic and also that our East Indian heritage predisposed me to estrogen dominance—which showed up as glaringly obvious in many of my close relatives and friends. I knew I was fighting an uphill battle against hormone dysregulation, but I was determined to find a better way.

I worked tirelessly to keep my own hormones in check, and I was successful. I was able to head off the symptoms that had plagued others in my family before they even started. I felt like I had cracked the code—I knew what foods to eat, what herbs to take, and how to maintain balance in my body. When I hit my perimenopausal years, I felt fully equipped to handle it. I figured I would sail through this stage of life without a hitch because I had done everything right. I knew how to manage symptoms, and I wasn't worried about hormonal havoc heading my way.

But then everything changed. A devastating car accident left me with a concussion, and suddenly, all the tools and knowledge I had relied on were no longer enough. My body went into a tailspin. Brain fog, fatigue, and anxiety took over. I didn't feel like myself. My periods became unbearably heavy—so much so that doctors were talking about transfusions. It was like my entire hormonal system had been thrown into chaos overnight. I began to research and found that concussions could disrupt hormones in profound ways, triggering a cascade of issues. The timing couldn't have been worse; I was already in the hormonally sensitive time of perimenopause, and the accident had only made things more volatile.

I knew I needed more than my usual remedies. I needed answers that I couldn't find in the usual places. I turned to saliva hormone panel testing, desperate to get a clear picture of what was going on inside my body. The results were eye-opening: my cortisol levels were almost non-existent, my estrogen and progesterone were completely out of sync, and my thyroid was barely keeping up. For someone who had spent her entire life managing health and balance, seeing those results was both shocking and humbling. I realized that even I, with all my knowledge, couldn't get the information I needed without proper testing.

That's when it hit me—I wasn't alone. So many women, just like me, were navigating hormone imbalances without the right tools or resources. I had to make this information and testing available to others, so they didn't have to struggle in the dark. I began incorporating comprehensive hormone testing into my wellness practice, not just for myself but for my clients too. It wasn't just about guessing what was wrong; it was about seeing the data and understanding the intricate dance of hormones at play. Armed with this knowledge, we could finally get to the root of the problem and find real solutions.

The transformation I experienced as a result of the right testing and proper therapies was nothing short of life-changing. With a targeted plan based on my test results, I slowly began to reclaim my health. My energy returned, my mind cleared, and I felt like myself again. The accident was a turning point, forcing me to seek out new tools and knowledge that I now share with everyone who walks through my door.

This journey taught me that no matter how much you know, sometimes life throws you a curveball, and you need more. You need data, you need insights, and you need a plan. My mission is to make sure no woman feels helpless in the face of hormonal chaos. With the right testing, the right guidance, and the right mindset, we can all find our way back to balance.

Join us as we explore together!

Darpan and Kathy

TABLE OF CONTENTS

CHAPTER 1

YOU ARE YOUR HORMONES

Imagine waking up every day feeling energized, focused, and in control. Your mood is stable, you sleep like a baby, and you rarely get sick. You have little to no aches, pains or other health issues, and you're more physically active than most of your friends.

Now, picture the opposite: fatigue, mood swings, insomnia, frequent infections, autoimmune or chronic health conditions, pain, and a sense of always being on edge.

The difference between these two realities often comes down to one powerful word: hormones. These tiny chemical messengers influence every aspect of our lives—from our energy levels and mental clarity to our immunity, pain levels, and even our personality.

You ARE your hormones.

Think about it: why are some people naturally happy while others struggle with mood swings? Why are some people full of energy while others feel perpetually tired? Why do some of us thrive as night owls while others are morning people? Yes, personality, mindset, and habits play a role, but at the core of it all are your hormones.

They influence everything from how well you sleep and how much energy you have to your ability to think clearly, feel happy, and jump out of bed in the morning. When you understand that your hormones influence every function in your body, it becomes clear: you ARE your hormones.

Hormones are like the conductors of an orchestra, coordinating the various sections to create a harmonious symphony. When they are in balance, life feels like a beautiful piece of music. But when they are out of sync, the result is a chaotic cacophony. Think about how your energy levels fluctuate. Cortisol, estrogen, progesterone, testosterone, DHEA, and your thyroid hormones are your body's natural regulators. When balanced, they keep you alert and ready to tackle your day. Out of whack? Say hello to chronic fatigue, mood swings, and feeling like you're losing control of your own body and mind.

Let's explore these key hormones and how they

influence us on a moment-to-moment basis.

Estrogen: Your Diva Hormone

Estrogen is primarily known for its role in the female reproductive system, but it plays a role in the health of both sexes. Balanced estrogen levels can boost mood, energy, and overall well-being. Too much estrogen, however, can lead to weight gain, menstrual problems, mood swings, and issues like fibroids, endometriosis, and cysts. In men, high estrogen can contribute to weight gain, particularly around the belly, and even lead to gynecomastia (enlarged breast tissue). Low estrogen levels can cause symptoms like fatigue, depression, and decreased libido, leading to issues with mood, vaginal dryness, and pain during intercourse.

Progesterone: Your “Calm Down” Companion

Progesterone works in tandem with estrogen to regulate the menstrual cycle and maintain pregnancy. It has a calming effect on the body, promoting better sleep and reducing anxiety. Low progesterone levels can lead to symptoms like anxiety, insomnia, and irregular menstrual cycles. Low progesterone can often cause women to feel like they’re on an emotional rollercoaster with no brakes. High levels of progesterone, although less common, can cause sleepiness, mood swings, and even dizziness. Progesterone is considered a "mother" hormone as it converts to testosterone, estrogen, and cortisol. This is why it is also important to consider not just the individual hormone levels but the ratio between them.

Testosterone: Your Vitality Booster

Testosterone is often associated with men, but it is crucial for women's health too. It helps maintain muscle mass, bone density, and libido. Low testosterone can present like a loss of vitality, as if the spark has gone out. In women, low testosterone can also result in a diminished sex drive, fatigue, hair loss, and muscle weakness. High levels of testosterone can lead to aggressive behavior, acne, and excessive hair growth in women, along with a higher risk of cardiovascular and fertility problems.

DHEA: The Unsung Hormone Hero

DHEA (dehydroepiandrosterone) is one of the most abundant hormones in the body and plays a crucial role in maintaining overall health. Produced by the adrenal glands, DHEA serves as a precursor to both estrogen and testosterone. It helps support immune function, maintain energy levels, and promote a sense of well-being. Despite its importance, DHEA often doesn't get the attention it deserves. When DHEA levels are optimal, you feel energized, resilient to stress, and generally well. However, too much DHEA can lead to issues such as oily skin, acne, and excessive hair growth in women. It might also cause aggressiveness and irritability. On the flip side, low DHEA levels can result in fatigue, low libido, and a decreased sense of well-being. It's not uncommon for people with low DHEA to feel perpetually exhausted and unable to cope with stress effectively.

Cortisol: The Stress Bufferer

Cortisol is often called the stress hormone, and for a good reason. It helps manage how your body uses carbohydrates, fats, and proteins. It helps reduce inflammation, control blood sugar levels, and regulate your sleep-wake cycle. But too much cortisol, often due to chronic stress, can lead to problems like weight gain, high blood pressure, and a weakened immune system. Imagine constantly feeling on edge, unable to relax, and seeing the physical toll it takes on your body. That's high cortisol at work. Too little cortisol can leave you feeling fatigued, weak, and even depressed. It's like trying to drive a car with no fuel—you just can't get going.

Insulin: The Sugar Regulator

Insulin, often overlooked in discussions about hormonal health, plays a critical role in managing blood sugar levels and directly impacts other hormones. When insulin is balanced, it helps regulate blood sugar, supports energy production, and keeps inflammation in check. However, when insulin levels are chronically high—often due to a diet high in refined sugars and processed foods—it can lead to insulin resistance, a precursor to type 2 diabetes. Insulin resistance doesn't just impact blood sugar; it can throw off your entire hormonal system, leading to weight gain, increased cortisol, and imbalances in estrogen and testosterone. The beauty of insulin is that it's one of the few hormones you have significant control over through diet and lifestyle. By eating balanced meals with adequate protein, healthy fats, and fiber, you can keep your blood sugar—and insulin levels—in check, positively influencing your overall hormonal balance.

Vitamin D: The Hormone in Disguise

Vitamin D, often referred to as the "sunshine vitamin," is actually more of a hormone than a vitamin, playing a pivotal role in regulating other hormones throughout the body. It influences the function of nearly every cell and helps modulate the immune system, reduce inflammation, and balance mood. Low levels of vitamin D are linked to a wide range of health issues, including hormonal imbalances, autoimmune conditions, and even depression. Despite its importance, vitamin D deficiency is incredibly common, affecting millions worldwide. Optimizing vitamin D levels is crucial for supporting your overall hormonal health; think of it as the hormone that sets the stage for all other hormones to perform their best. Regular sunlight exposure, vitamin D-rich foods, and supplementation when necessary can help ensure your levels are where they need to be for optimal health.

These hormones affect not only your physical health but also your mental and emotional well-being. When they are out of balance, you might feel like you can't "get it together." You might wonder why you can't think clearly, why you're always tired, or why you're in a perpetual bad mood. Or maybe your anxiety continues to creep up at the most inopportune times. It's not your fault—it's your hormones. Too often, we've been told that many of these symptoms are normal, especially as we age, but common and normal are not the same thing.

I want to stop here for a minute and have you think about the guilt or shame that often accompanies the downside to hormonal imbalance. You berate yourself for not being more productive, for snapping at loved ones (or strangers!), or for not having the energy to exercise. On one hand, you are judged for your inability to do and be all that is expected of you, but on the other hand, society tends to dismiss these symptoms as just part of getting older or being "hormonal." Eyes are rolled, the term "Karen" is thrown around, and concerns (legitimate or not) are brushed off as "PMS" or "menopause."

This is interesting, because it shows us that there IS a general awareness of how hormones impact mood and personality—but the level of judgment and dismissiveness remains high. Hormones do not in any way give someone license to be rude, abusive or in a perpetual bad mood, but if we assume that the majority of people desire to be happy, productive, and patient, maybe we can start to see that in most cases, something deeper is going on that is contributing to these less desirable personality traits. It's crucial to recognize these symptoms are signals from your body that something is off balance. They are not a reflection of your willpower or your character; they are biological signals that need attention.

To go from hormone havoc to hormone bliss,

the first thing you need to do is understand the monthly rhythm and cycle of our hormones. If I asked nine women out of ten, they probably could not explain what is happening during each stage of their cycle, but understanding these phases is crucial for harnessing the power of your hormones.

Let's break down how your hormones guide you through the month, and how these shifts affect your energy, focus, and productivity.

The menstrual cycle is much more than just a monthly occurrence; it's a powerful rhythm that influences every aspect of your life, from your energy levels and motivation to your mood and productivity. By tuning into this cycle, you can start to understand why you might feel on top of the world one week and sluggish the next. Instead of fighting against these natural fluctuations, embracing them can help you harness your full potential.

Let's start with the follicular phase, which begins right after your period ends. During this time, estrogen levels start to rise, leading to an increase in energy, motivation, and mental clarity. This phase is often characterized by a natural inclination towards being more active, both physically and mentally. You might find that this is when you're most eager to hit the gym, take on new projects, or socialize with friends. Your brain is sharper, your mood is brighter, and your confidence is higher.

This is the time to plan, strategize, and kickstart those tasks that require creativity and enthusiasm. Women often report feeling more adventurous and ready to tackle challenges during this phase, making it the perfect time to set goals and start new initiatives.

As you approach ovulation, around day 14 of your cycle, your estrogen and testosterone levels peak. This is when you're likely to feel your absolute best. You're sociable, energetic, and at the top of your game. It's no coincidence that many women find themselves more outgoing and charismatic during this phase; your body is biologically primed to be at its most vibrant. This is the ideal time for networking, giving presentations, or engaging in any activity that requires confidence and communication skills. Your productivity is likely at its highest, and you may notice that tasks that seemed daunting just a week ago are now being completed with ease.

However, after ovulation, you enter the luteal phase, in which progesterone takes the lead. This phase is often misunderstood because it comes with a natural slowdown. Energy levels may begin to dip, and you might feel a shift towards introspection and hibernation. This is not a time to push yourself to match the high-energy output of the follicular phase, but rather a time to focus on completing tasks and winding down. It's common for women to feel frustrated during this phase, especially if they try to maintain the same pace they had during the follicular phase. You might find yourself upset that you "didn't accomplish anything all week." This is your hormones at work, and it's perfectly normal.

Recognizing these patterns of high motivation and sociability during the follicular phase, contrasted with the more introspective and slower-paced luteal phase, can be life-changing. Instead of feeling guilty for not being consistently productive, you can start to plan your life around these natural cycles. By aligning your activities, diet, and self-care routines with your hormonal phases, you can maximize your well-being and achieve a more balanced, fulfilling life.

Understanding your hormonal cycle isn't just about recognizing the highs and lows in your energy and motivation—it's also about acknowledging that women's hormonal rhythms are fundamentally different from men's. While women operate on a 28-day cycle that influences mood, energy, and productivity throughout the month, men's hormones follow a 24-hour cycle, allowing them to have relatively consistent energy and focus day after day. This daily cycle of testosterone peaks in the morning and gradually declines throughout the day, allowing men to maintain a steady level of productivity and performance that aligns perfectly with the "hustle" and "seize the day" culture that dominates high-performance and motivational spaces.

For women, this one-size-fits-all approach can be frustrating and unsustainable. The constant push to grind without breaks, hustle harder, and maintain peak performance every single day often runs counter to the natural ebbs and flows of the female hormonal cycle. Many women find themselves depleted, burnt out, or feeling like they can't keep up when trying to adopt these "no excuses" mentalities.

It's not that women aren't capable of hustling just as hard or achieving the same level of success as men—it's that our productivity doesn't follow the same daily rhythm. By tuning into the ebbs and flows of your 28-day cycle, you can capitalize on the high-energy phases to push forward and use the slower phases for reflection and strategic planning, allowing you to work smarter, not harder. Understanding these cycles empowers women to be just as productive, successful, and resilient as men, but in a way that honors their unique hormonal rhythms rather than working against them.

By embracing your natural cycles, you can plan your most challenging tasks during high-energy phases and allow for rest and reflection when your body calls for it. This approach not only boosts productivity but also sustains it, helping you achieve your goals without the burnout that comes from forcing yourself into a mold that was never designed for you. Success doesn't have to come at the expense of your health, but can be achieved by working in harmony with your body's natural design.

There are no accidents in nature. Everything from the tides of the oceans to the migration patterns of animals follows a rhythm, a natural order that has existed since the beginning of time. And when you take a closer look, you'll notice a fascinating pattern: the average length of a woman's menstrual cycle is almost identical to the cycle of the moon, both lasting about 28 days.

This connection is not coincidence. Ancient

cultures observed this powerful parallel, noting that while men were "ruled by the sun" with its consistent 24-hour cycle representing linear productivity and daily renewal, women were deeply connected to the moon. For thousands of years, the moon has been a symbol of feminine energy, transformation, and renewal. In cultures of the ancient Greeks and the Chinese, the moon was often associated with goddesses and feminine power, representing the cycle of birth, growth, decay, and rebirth.

In many Indigenous cultures, like some of the First Nations people of North America, women's cycles were seen as sacred and aligned with the phases of the moon—embodying the waxing and waning of the moon's phases.

This concept of being "ruled by the moon" reflects an inherent wisdom that we've largely lost in our modern world. Today, we live disconnected from the natural environment that once shaped our rhythms. Artificial lights, screens, and constant exposure to technology have severed our ties to nature's cycles. But some believe that if we were to live without the interference of artificial light, screens, and the endless noise of modern life, our bodies would naturally sync with the moon's cycle.

New moon would coincide with menstruation, and ovulation would occur around the full moon. During the waxing moon, women would feel the rising energy of the follicular phase, while the waning moon would mirror the introspection and slowing down of the luteal phase.

Imagine a world where women's cycles are honored in alignment with these lunar phases. During the new moon, a time of darkness and renewal, women would be in their menstrual phase—a time for rest, reflection, and turning inward. The waxing moon, symbolizing growth and expansion, aligns with the follicular phase when energy is building, creativity is high, and new projects are ready to take flight. As the moon becomes full, a woman's cycle reaches its peak with ovulation, a time of vibrancy, sociability, and maximum energy. Finally, the waning moon brings a gentle descent into the luteal phase, where energy starts to wane, reflection becomes key, and it's time to wrap up and prepare for a new cycle.

Bringing this ancient wisdom back into our modern lives isn't about following rigid rules or adding more pressure; it's about reconnecting with the natural rhythms that have always been a part of us. Even if your cycle isn't perfectly aligned with the moon right now, simply being aware of these connections can help you understand your body's signals on a deeper level. And this connection isn't just for menstruating women; menopausal women, who no longer have their own cycles to guide them, can also turn to the moon. By observing the moon phases, you can chart your more productive days and recognize when it's time to slow down, just as a woman with a menstrual cycle does.

Think of this as a way to bring the wisdom of the past into the present. By syncing your life with these ancient rhythms, you honor the deep, powerful connection between your body and nature. Whether you're planning your most ambitious projects during the full moon or setting intentions during the new moon, you can tap into this cyclical wisdom to guide your energy and focus. Embracing this concept allows us to reconnect with a part of ourselves that the modern world often overlooks, reminding us that we are not separate from nature but an integral part of its beautiful, rhythmic dance.

CHAPTER 2

HORMONES UNLEASHED: THE ROLLERCOASTER RIDE OF YOUR LIFE

Buckle up, because when your hormones decide to go rogue, life feels like you're strapped into a rollercoaster that never stops. One moment you're on top of the world, and the next, you're plummeting into an abyss of anxiety, brain fog, and tears over a commercial for cat food. It's not just you; it's your hormones running the show, turning your body into a funhouse of unpredictable twists and turns. And if you think your hormones are just doing their own thing, think again—these little chemical messengers are all interconnected, working together in an elaborate web that, when tangled, can make you feel like you've lost control.

This chapter will take you on a deep dive into the intricate web of how everything in our body is interconnected and how external factors like the environment and diet contribute to hormonal chaos.

Hormones don't operate in isolation. They interact with each other in a complex, delicate balance. When one hormone is out of balance, it can set off a domino effect that impacts the entire system. For instance, did you know that high estrogen levels can negatively impact the thyroid, slowing metabolism and causing symptoms like fatigue and weight gain? This one simple example highlights the complex interplay between hormones.

Another example is the relationship between insulin and cortisol. Insulin is a hormone that regulates blood sugar levels. When you eat, insulin is released to help your cells absorb glucose for energy. However, if you're constantly stressed your body remains in a state of heightened alert. This can lead to insulin resistance, meaning your cells no longer respond to insulin effectively. As a result, your body produces more insulin to compensate, leading to higher blood sugar levels and, eventually, if unaddressed, conditions like type 2 diabetes.

External factors also play a significant role in hormonal balance. Environmental toxins and pollutants can act as endocrine disruptors, interfering with hormone production and function. Toxins found in plastics, personal care products, and even some food packaging can mimic or block hormones, leading to imbalances. For example, bisphenol A (BPA), a common chemical in plastics, can mimic estrogen in the body, leading to elevated estrogen levels and a host of related symptoms like weight gain, mood swings, and reproductive issues.

And it's not just plastics. The bathroom cabinet and cleaning supplies under your sink are full of potential hormonal landmines. Parabens and phthalates are hiding in your shampoos, lotions, and even that "fresh scent" air freshener. These chemicals act like hormonal saboteurs, messing with testosterone and estrogen levels. The fix? Start swapping your everyday products for cleaner, non-toxic options.

Diet is another critical factor. Processed foods, additives, and artificial ingredients can wreak havoc on your hormones. Diets high in sugar and refined carbohydrates can spike insulin levels and lead to insulin resistance. Meanwhile, trans fats and artificial preservatives can disrupt the balance of hormones by causing inflammation and oxidative stress. A diet lacking in essential nutrients like omega-3 fatty acids can further exacerbate hormonal imbalances, making it harder for your body to produce and regulate hormones effectively.

Lifestyle factors also contribute to hormonal disruptions. Lack of sleep, for instance, can elevate cortisol levels and suppress melatonin production, disrupting your sleep-wake cycle. Inadequate physical activity can lead to poor insulin sensitivity and weight gain, further stressing your hormonal balance. Chronic stress, whether from work, relationships, or other sources, keeps your body in a state of constant fight-or-flight, flooding your system with cortisol and throwing other hormones out of balance.

Let's dive into some of the most common players in hormonal imbalances—those familiar faces that keep showing up in almost every hormone profile I look at.

Estrogen dominance is one of the most common issues I see in my practice, affecting women from the onset of puberty and beyond. If not addressed, it can lead to conditions like fibroids, endometriosis, worsening PMS, polyps, and heavy, flooding periods. At its core, estrogen dominance happens when there's too much estrogen relative to progesterone, creating a hormonal imbalance that can trigger everything from weight gain, mood swings, and irregular menstrual cycles to fibroids, endometriosis and infertility.

But the story doesn't end there. Estrogen's impact goes beyond these symptoms, deeply intertwining with thyroid function. High estrogen levels increase thyroid-binding globulin, a protein that binds to thyroid hormones and reduces their availability in the body. You're tired, constipated, gaining weight, and if that's not enough, poor gut health reabsorbs the extra estrogen, feeding the vicious cycle. It's a hormonal Groundhog Day you just can't escape.

The effects of estrogen dominance are not just physical; they reach into the emotional and psychological realms as well. Anxiety, irritability, and depression are common companions of this hormonal imbalance, especially during the premenstrual phase when estrogen levels fluctuate more dramatically. For many women, these emotional symptoms start young, leading to mood swings, heightened sensitivity, and a sense of being overwhelmed—feelings that are often dismissed as "normal" teenage moodiness but are, in fact, signs of deeper hormonal issues.

Next up, Polycystic Ovary Syndrome (PCOS)—a hormonal circus act that's part testosterone overload, part insulin resistance, and 100% frustrating. PCOS doesn't just mess with your period; it's the gift that keeps on giving with symptoms like weight gain, acne, and hair growth in places you'd rather not discuss. It's estimated that 1 in 10 women has PCOS, but it's not just a reproductive issue. It's a full-body condition that throws off everything from your metabolism to your mental health. Beyond the physical symptoms, PCOS can feel like a relentless uphill battle, especially when the weight doesn't budge, even when you're eating kale and doing all the right things. It's not you; it's your hormones turning the odds against you.

High testosterone in women might sound like a free pass to extra strength and stamina, but trust me, it's not. It's all the symptoms of PCOS and a deep-seated irritability that can make even the calmest among us feel like flipping tables. And low testosterone? Equally as frustrating, but in a different way. We're talking fatigue, muscle loss, and a libido that packed its bags and left town. Low testosterone doesn't just zap your energy; it steals your motivation, your zest for life, and your ability to feel like, well, you.

Then there's cortisol—the notorious stress hormone that's supposed to save the day but often overstays its welcome. Mainstream medicine only acknowledges cortisol when it's at the extreme ends, like in Cushing's or Addison's disease, but the reality is that adrenal health exists on a spectrum.

High cortisol makes you feel like you're living with a perpetual alarm bell going off. Weight gain around the belly, high blood pressure, frequent colds—it's like your body's stuck in a never-ending fight-or-flight mode. And low cortisol, often labeled "adrenal fatigue" even though mainstream docs love to say it's not a thing, leaves you dragging through the day with zero energy, no stress tolerance, and a sense of overwhelm at the smallest hiccup. It's not just tired; it's can't-get-off-the-couch, can't-handle-life tired.

The broad spectrum of hormonal imbalances—from estrogen dominance to PCOS, high and low testosterone, and fluctuating cortisol levels—can have profound effects on physical, emotional, and psychological health. Understanding the root causes and addressing these imbalances is key to regaining control and improving overall well-being.

Recognizing these patterns and understanding the interplay between hormones and lifestyle factors is the first step in regaining control. It's not about blaming yourself for feeling off balance; it's about acknowledging that many of these issues stem from factors within and beyond our control. By addressing these factors—through better diet, appropriate supplementation, and lifestyle adjustments—we can start to bring our hormones back into harmony.

I can't tell you how many times clients come to consult with me and they feel like they're losing their minds, only to be told by their doctors that their hormone levels are "normal." But here's the thing: "normal" doesn't mean optimal, and it sure doesn't mean you're feeling your best.

This is where a holistic perspective is crucial. Traditional medical tests often fall short in detecting subtle imbalances that can have a significant impact on your health. Normal ranges are broad and don't account for individual variability. Just because your results fall within the normal range doesn't mean your hormones are functioning optimally. The levels you need to feel your best are likely different from the standardized "norm" you're compared to.

So, what do you do? You advocate for yourself. You find a healthcare provider who actually listens, who sees you as a person, not just a collection of lab results. Someone who understands that if you feel off, then something is off. Trust your gut—you know your body better than anyone.

The right provider will look at the whole picture, not just the pieces that fit neatly into the "normal" category.

And here's the good news: hormonal imbalances don't have to be your life sentence. These aren't just random symptoms you have to live with; they're red flags from your body waving frantically to get your attention. They're not here to ruin your life; they're here to tell you that something needs to change. When you start paying attention to these signals and taking steps to address them, you begin to take back control. This journey might feel like a rollercoaster at times, but with awareness and action, you can smooth out the ride and enjoy a more balanced, vibrant life.

CHAPTER 3

PMS SOS: UNDERSTANDING THE MONTHLY MADNESS

You've probably heard it a million times: "PMS is normal; it's just something women have to put up with."

Well, I'm here to tell you that this is complete bunk. The reality is, your period should come and go without hijacking your life or turning you into a moody mess. The narrative that PMS is unavoidable and "just part of being a woman" is not only wrong—it's holding us back from understanding our bodies and taking control of our hormonal health.

Hormonal issues and menstrual problems have become increasingly common in today's world, thanks to modern lifestyle factors, environmental toxins, chronic stress, and changes in our diets. Historically, there's little evidence to suggest that widespread menstrual or hormonal disorders were as prevalent as they are now. It's not just that these issues were not talked about or considered taboo—they were most likely far less common. The sharp rise we see today indicates that what was once considered an unusual disruption in hormonal health has, unfortunately, become the norm.

What we do know is that understanding and managing your hormones can make many of these common monthly symptoms disappear. By exploring the intricate dance between estrogen and progesterone and learning how to balance these hormones, it is possible to greatly reduce the symptoms of PMS.

In this chapter, we'll delve into the specifics of PMS, the roles of estrogen and progesterone, and how imbalances between these hormones can create the storm of symptoms that we now deem to be a normal part of life for most women.

PMS, or premenstrual syndrome, is a common condition that affects up to 75% of menstruating women. It encompasses a wide range of symptoms that occur in the luteal phase of the menstrual cycle, typically one week before menstruation begins. These symptoms can include mood swings, bloating, headaches, breast tenderness, fatigue, irritability, and anxiety. The severity of PMS can vary greatly from woman to woman, with some experiencing mild discomfort and others being significantly impacted in their daily lives.

The root cause of PMS lies in the natural fluctuations of hormones that occur throughout the menstrual cycle. In the second half of the cycle, after ovulation, progesterone levels rise to prepare the body for a potential pregnancy. If pregnancy does not occur, progesterone levels drop sharply, leading to menstruation. It's this drop in progesterone that can put women into a more significant estrogen-dominant state. It is this relative imbalance between estrogen and progesterone that contributes to the symptoms of PMS.

Estrogen dominance is a major culprit behind the symptoms of PMS. It's like that one friend who's great fun at the party but overstays their welcome—loud, bossy, and impossible to ignore. High estrogen levels can disrupt mood, cause water retention, and make your breasts feel so tender they can't even stand the touch of your own clothes.

Estrogen dominance not only disrupts mood and physical comfort but also extends its influence to other critical hormonal systems, including the thyroid. The interplay between estrogen and the thyroid is not insignificant. As previously mentioned, high estrogen levels can bind thyroid hormones and reduce their availability to the body. This can slow down the thyroid, contributing to fatigue, constipation, and other symptoms of a sluggish metabolism.

I sometimes get asked, "If estrogen is often associated with symptoms like brain fog, irritability, and anxiety, why do most women feel better during the first half of their cycle when estrogen levels are higher than progesterone?" The answer to this question lies in the unique role estrogen plays during the follicular phase. As estrogen rises during this time, it exerts a positive influence on mood, energy, and mental clarity. Estrogen stimulates neurotransmitters like serotonin and dopamine, which are linked to feelings of well-being, motivation, and sharp mental focus. This is why many women feel more vibrant, optimistic, and energized as they move through the first half of their cycle.

In the follicular phase, estrogen is high but balanced with other hormones like testosterone, creating a harmonious hormonal environment that promotes confidence, sociability, and increased libido. This balance allows women to feel at their best—both mentally and physically.

It's crucial to differentiate between the high, balanced estrogen of the follicular phase and estrogen dominance, in which estrogen is disproportionately high relative to progesterone later in the cycle. Estrogen dominance often rears its head when estrogen is out of balance, leading to those dreaded symptoms like brain fog and anxiety. But during the first half of the cycle, estrogen is in its sweet spot, fueling not just the body but also the mind, making women feel alive, focused, and ready to take on the world.

But estrogen is only one side of the coin. Low progesterone levels can exacerbate PMS symptoms. Progesterone has a calming effect on the body, promoting relaxation and sleep. It also helps to counterbalance the effects of estrogen. When progesterone levels are low, the body loses this calming influence, leading to increased anxiety, irritability, and difficulty sleeping. Furthermore, low progesterone can contribute to heavy menstrual bleeding and irregular cycles, as it is essential for regulating the menstrual cycle and maintaining the uterine lining.

If you are experiencing symptoms of PMS, this is a sign that your progesterone levels are too low or are dropping too far too fast at the end of your cycle. Thankfully, we have ways to mitigate this problem and restore natural balance.

The relationship between progesterone and cortisol adds another layer of complexity, particularly when a woman is under stress. Progesterone is not only crucial for reproductive health but also serves as the precursor, or "mother hormone," of cortisol, the body's main stress hormone. When progesterone levels are low, your body faces a critical choice: use the available progesterone to help keep you calm, balanced, and reduce PMS symptoms or convert it into cortisol to keep you alive.

Spoiler alert: survival always wins.

The truth is, your body can function, albeit poorly, with low progesterone—you might feel irritable, anxious, and fatigued, but you'll survive. However, without adequate cortisol, survival isn't possible; cortisol is essential for managing stress, maintaining blood pressure, and keeping your body's systems running. This is why your body will always prioritize cortisol production over maintaining optimal progesterone levels, even if it means sacrificing your mood and well-being in the process.

This process, often referred to as the "progesterone steal," diverts progesterone into the production of cortisol, leaving less available for its calming and regulatory roles. As a result, women under chronic stress may find their PMS symptoms worsen because the body continuously sacrifices progesterone to meet cortisol demands. This creates a vicious cycle in which stress not only disrupts overall hormonal balance but also exacerbates the very symptoms of irritability, anxiety, and sleep disturbances that progesterone would normally help mitigate.

The impact of this hormonal tug-of-war doesn't stop at PMS. If you're already dealing with chronic health conditions, autoimmune disorders, or chronic pain, the progesterone steal doesn't just make PMS worse—it throws gas on an already raging fire. Many women with conditions like lupus, rheumatoid arthritis, or fibromyalgia find their symptoms flare during the luteal phase when progesterone is most needed. The stress of managing these conditions pulls even more progesterone into cortisol production, leaving your body without the hormonal support it desperately needs.

This is why you might notice your pain or autoimmune symptoms intensifying right before your period. Without enough of this crucial "mother hormone" to go around, the body's ability to regulate immune function, pain perception, and inflammation is compromised, leading to intensified symptoms and making these health conditions harder to manage during these critical hormonal windows.

So, what can you do when PMS feels like it's running your life? How can we bring balance back to this hormonally sensitive time of the month?

Traditionally, the primary option offered to women for managing PMS has been the birth control pill. While birth control pills can sometimes help to alleviate symptoms in the short term, they are often only masking the real problem and can create additional issues in the long term. The mechanism of the birth control pill involves suppressing the body's natural hormones and offering synthetic hormones in their place. This suppression of natural hormone production can lead to a range of side effects and long-term health implications.

One of the significant drawbacks of birth control pills and other forms of synthetic HRT is their impact on nutrient levels in the body. HRT can deplete essential nutrients, including B vitamins and magnesium, which are critical for energy production, mood regulation, and overall health. A deficiency in these nutrients can lead to fatigue, mood swings, and other symptoms that can further complicate hormonal imbalances.

Moreover, many women have issues with the synthetic progestins found in birth control pills. Unlike bio-identical progesterone, which is chemically identical to the hormone produced by the body, synthetic progestins can have different and often more severe side effects. Common side effects of synthetic progestins include irritability, depression, and anxiety. These mental health issues can significantly impact a woman's quality of life and are often not adequately addressed by healthcare providers.

It has been my experience that most women are not informed of the potential side effects or long-term impacts of synthetic HRT use. I can't tell you how many times I have heard of women starting on the birth control pill, only to see a dramatic downturn in their mental health. Then, instead of going off the pill, they are prescribed antidepressants or anti-anxiety medications to help them deal with the side effects.

This is a problem as many women end up on both the birth control pill and antidepressants for years or decades—and don't get me started on how we are putting young teens on the pill when their bodies are just beginning to learn how to cycle and ovulate. Then they stay on the pill into their thirties and then can't understand why they can't get pregnant.

Bio-identical hormones offer a more natural alternative for hormone replacement. Bio-identical progesterone can help balance estrogen levels and alleviate PMS symptoms without the common side effects associated with synthetic progestins. Women using bio-identical hormones often report fewer side effects and a better overall sense of well-being. We'll be doing a deep dive on the pros and cons of bio-identical hormones as well as the best vitamins, minerals, and herbs to help balance hormones in chapter 9.

The reality is, most women don't actually need added hormones to balance their hormones. Many of the symptoms of PMS can be mitigated through diet, lifestyle, and proper supplementation. Added hormones should rarely be the very first intervention. From a holistic perspective, there are many natural remedies and lifestyle changes that can help balance estrogen and progesterone levels and alleviate PMS symptoms.

First and foremost, diet plays a crucial role in hormonal balance. Eating a diet rich in whole, unprocessed foods can support hormone health. Cruciferous vegetables like broccoli, cauliflower, and Brussels sprouts contain compounds that help the body metabolize estrogen more effectively. Incorporating healthy fats, such as those found in avocados, nuts, and seeds, can support progesterone production. Sources of protein—both animal and vegetarian—are essential for proper nutrient intake and optimal hormonal health. Additionally, reducing sugar and refined carbohydrates can help stabilize blood sugar levels and prevent insulin resistance, which can exacerbate hormonal imbalances.

Something else you may want to try is seed cycling, a simple yet powerful practice that can help balance hormones naturally throughout your cycle. Seed cycling involves consuming specific seeds during the different phases of your menstrual cycle to promote estrogen and progesterone balance. During the follicular phase (Day 1 to ovulation), which is when estrogen is dominant, consume 1 tablespoon each of ground flaxseed and pumpkin seeds daily. Flaxseeds contain lignans that help regulate estrogen levels, while pumpkin seeds are rich in zinc, which supports the healthy release of progesterone later in the cycle. Other seeds that you can also use during this phase are chia seeds or hemp seeds.

As you move into the luteal phase (ovulation

to the start of your next period), switch to 1 tablespoon each of sunflower and sesame seeds daily. Sunflower seeds are high in vitamin E and selenium, which support progesterone production, while sesame seeds contain lignans that help block excess estrogen. This cycling of seeds can provide the body with the right nutrients at the right time, encouraging a more balanced hormonal landscape and alleviating symptoms like PMS, irregular cycles, and mood swings.

Seed cycling is a gentle, natural way to work with your body's hormonal rhythms and can be a valuable addition to your overall hormone-balancing strategy. If you do not have a regular cycle, you can use the phases of the moon to determine your seed cycling routine. Days 1-14 (new moon to full moon), eat pumpkin seeds and flax seeds. Days 15-28 (full moon to new moon), eat sunflower seeds and sesame seeds.

Exercise is another powerful tool for managing hormonal imbalances, but it's important to tailor your workouts to your cycle. Remember, during the follicular phase, your body is more resilient to stress, making it the perfect time for high-intensity workouts like HIIT, running, and strength training.

However, during the luteal phase, when your body's demand for progesterone is high, intense exercise can add unnecessary stress, spiking cortisol and stealing from available progesterone. This is when it's best to switch to lower-impact activities like yoga, Pilates, rebounding, and walking to support progesterone and keep cortisol in balance, helping you feel more aligned with your body's needs.

Stress management is essential for maintaining hormonal balance and reducing PMS symptoms. Practices like mindfulness meditation, deep breathing exercises, and spending time in nature can help lower stress levels and support hormonal health. In addition, adequate sleep is crucial, as poor sleep can further disrupt hormone balance and intensify PMS symptoms.

As you can see, there are numerous strategies within your control that can significantly reduce PMS symptoms and restore hormonal balance naturally. From adjusting your diet and exercise routine to managing stress and exploring natural supplements, you have the power to make meaningful changes. You don't have to approach this time of the month with fear, anxiety, or the sense that it's something you simply have to endure. You can take proactive steps to support your body's natural rhythms and create a more harmonious hormonal environment.

It's time to rewrite the story you've been told—that PMS is just your cross to bear and that the only solution is a prescription. Instead, you can empower yourself with knowledge and natural strategies to balance your hormones, reduce your symptoms, and get back to feeling like yourself. You're not powerless. You can turn the tide on PMS and regain control of your body, your mood, and your life.

CHAPTER 4

MENOPAUSE, MOOD SWINGS, AND MUFFIN TOPS

Menopause is like nature's unexpected plot twist—a time when your body decides to flip the script, leaving you wondering who's really in charge. One minute, you're cruising through life, and the next, you're sweating through your sheets at 2 a.m., snapping at loved ones or staring down an ever-growing muffin top in the mirror. It's as if your body has decided to test you in ways you never saw coming.

For many women, menopause is a time of desperation and frustration. For the unprepared, hormonal shifts during this phase can turn life upside down, but when you understand the source of these symptoms, you can take action, both well before the perimenopausal years and also during or after them to reduce symptoms and improve your total health.

This chapter will explore the hormonal shifts that occur during menopause, focusing on the roles of the adrenals, cortisol, and DHEA, and provide strategies for managing this significant life transition.

Menopause is officially defined as the point when a woman has not had a menstrual period for 12 consecutive months. The average age of menopause in North America is 51, but the transition can start much earlier. Perimenopause, the period leading up to menopause, typically begins in a woman's 40s and can last anywhere from a few months to over a decade. During perimenopause, hormonal fluctuations become more pronounced, leading to symptoms such as irregular periods, hot flashes, night sweats, mood swings, and weight gain. Postmenopause refers to the time after menopause has occurred when symptoms may ease, but the risk for certain health conditions, like osteoporosis and cardiovascular disease, increases.

Menopausal experiences vary widely among women, with symptoms ranging from barely noticeable to severely disruptive. Research shows that about 20% of women experience extreme menopausal symptoms, such as intense hot flashes, night sweats, mood swings, and sleep disturbances that significantly impact their quality of life. Approximately 60% of women have moderate symptoms that are bothersome but manageable, including mild to moderate hot flashes and occasional sleep issues, while the remaining 20% report minimal to no symptoms, experiencing little discomfort during menopause.

Due to the severity of their symptoms, around 30-40% of women seek medical intervention, including hormone replacement therapy (HRT) or other medications, to manage their menopause-related challenges. This reliance on pharmaceutical support underscores the significant impact that severe menopausal symptoms can have on women's daily lives .

The drama of menopause centers around a steep drop in estrogen and progesterone—two hormones that have been your trusty sidekicks through the reproductive years. As the ovaries wind down their hormone production, the adrenals step up as backup, but they're not exactly star players. These tiny glands, perched on top of your kidneys, are now responsible for producing small amounts of estrogen and progesterone, along with cortisol, your body's primary stress hormone. If your adrenals are already taxed from years of chronic stress or poor lifestyle choices, their ability to compensate is limited, leaving you running on fumes.

This issue is compounded by the phenomenon of "progesterone stealing," which we discussed in detail in chapter 3. During menopause, this becomes an even bigger problem because the adrenals are now the primary source of progesterone. When stress is high, the body prioritizes cortisol production over progesterone, depleting an already limited supply. Dysregulated levels of cortisol can magnify menopausal symptoms, interfere with sleep, increase anxiety and depression, and contribute to weight gain, particularly around the abdomen—the so-called "muffin top." Cortisol promotes the storage of visceral fat, increasing the risk of metabolic syndrome and cardiovascular disease.

For many women, this dynamic leads to a confusing hormonal landscape: despite having low overall estrogen levels, they remain in a state of estrogen dominance relative to progesterone. This imbalance can cause symptoms like hot flashes, mood swings, and stubborn weight gain. It's crucial to understand that even with declining estrogen, the body's stress response can drive a persistent state of hormonal imbalance, making menopausal symptoms more severe and challenging to manage.

This is why, even though estrogen levels are generally low during perimenopause and menopause, simply adding estrogen as part of hormone replacement therapy (HRT) without carefully balancing it with adequate progesterone can worsen symptoms. When estrogen is introduced without adequate progesterone, it can amplify the state of estrogen dominance that persists even in low-estrogen environments. This imbalance can lead to intensified symptoms, leaving many women feeling worse rather than better.

Considering this delicate estrogen to progesterone ratio is crucial to avoid further tipping the scales and to support a more harmonious transition through menopause. This underscores the importance of personalized care and targeted strategies that consider the full hormonal picture, not just a single hormone in isolation.

Another crucial hormone during this transition is DHEA (dehydroepiandrosterone). DHEA is a precursor hormone produced by the adrenal glands, which the body can convert into testosterone and estrogen. It plays a significant role in overall vitality, energy levels, and stress management. As women approach menopause,

DHEA levels typically decline and supplementation may be warranted. However, because DHEA also converts into testosterone and estrogen, any supplementation needs to be managed with care and regular saliva hormone testing.

Everything previously discussed for managing PMS symptoms applies equally to perimenopausal and menopausal symptoms, as the overall goal remains the same: managing stress and maintaining a good ratio of progesterone to estrogen. Lifestyle modifications are essential for navigating menopause smoothly.

A common pattern I see is high-achieving, Type A women in their 50s who are accustomed to pushing themselves to the limit, with back-to-back spinning classes seven days a week, trying to outwork the stubborn weight that refuses to budge.

The thing is, when it comes to weight loss, what used to work in your 30s and 40s no longer does, and the intense workouts that once gave you that endorphin high are now revving up your body's need for cortisol. High-intensity, non-stop activity signals to your body that you're under constant stress, which only further drives up cortisol levels. This, in turn, leads to weight gain, particularly around the middle, and leaves you feeling more fatigued, burnt out, and frustrated than ever.

It seems counterintuitive, but to lose weight and feel your best during perimenopause and menopause, you often need to slow down instead of pushing harder. High-intensity workouts and a constantly on-the-go lifestyle force your body to prioritize cortisol production at the expense of other hormones like progesterone. Shifting to lower-impact activities—like yoga, Pilates, rebounding, or even taking long walks—helps calm your nervous system, balance cortisol, and preserve the delicate hormonal balance your body craves during this transition. Think of it as a more sustainable, gentler approach that nurtures rather than depletes. Slowing down doesn't mean giving up; it's about working with your body, not against it, to achieve the results you want.

Adequate sleep also plays a critical role; focusing on good sleep hygiene, creating a calming bedtime routine, and avoiding stimulants before bed can significantly improve sleep quality, reduce night sweats, and alleviate mood swings, making the menopausal transition much more manageable.

In addition to lifestyle changes, hormone replacement therapy (HRT) can be considered for managing severe menopausal symptoms. HRT involves supplementing the body with the missing hormones to alleviate symptoms. However, the goal should not be to have a 60-year-old with the hormones of a 20-year-old. Less is more when it comes to hormone therapy. The more we can do without hormones, the better.

Navigating menopause also requires more than just physical adjustments—it's about setting realistic expectations and managing your mental load. This transition can be a time of intense physical and emotional change, and it's okay to slow down and make space for yourself. Menopause often coincides with other life stressors, like juggling a career, managing a household, raising kids, or caring for aging parents. The more you can simplify, delegate, and let go of unrealistic expectations, the smoother your ride will be.

This is a season of life that asks for grace, patience, and a willingness to let go of what no longer serves you. Cut yourself some slack, reduce your commitments where you can, and lean on your support system. Menopause doesn't have to be a time of suffering—it's a powerful opportunity to reset, reprioritize, and embrace a new phase of life with wisdom and self-compassion.

Remember, your hormonal health isn't just about what's happening in your body—it's about your overall quality of life. You deserve to feel good, have energy, and maintain a positive outlook during this transition. Menopause isn't a punishment; it's a natural process that can be managed with the right tools and mindset. By taking proactive steps, you can transform your experience, reclaim your vitality, and redefine what it means to thrive during menopause.

This time of life should be about more than just surviving menopause—it's about learning to thrive in this new chapter. It's about understanding your body's changing needs and making adjustments that support your health, happiness, and well-being. With the right knowledge and a proactive approach, you can turn menopause from a time of dread into a time of empowerment and newfound freedom.

CHAPTER 5

UNDERSTANDING ANDROGENS: YOUR INNER WONDER WOMAN

If you've ever felt the surge of energy, the sudden burst of confidence, or the urge to take on the world, you've experienced the power of androgens. While often typecast as "male hormones," androgens like testosterone and DHEA are essential players in women's health, too. These hormones are the secret sauce behind muscle tone, libido, and that inner spark that makes you feel strong and capable. They are the unsung heroes that fuel your drive, courage, and resilience—the very traits that help you embody your inner Wonder Woman.

Before diving into this next key aspect of hormonal health, let's briefly recap some of the most important points we've covered so far. We've explored the powerful influence of hormones like estrogen and progesterone, highlighting how their delicate balance is essential for managing PMS, perimenopause, and menopause.

We've discussed the impact of cortisol and the phenomenon of progesterone stealing, emphasizing the importance of managing stress to support overall hormonal harmony.

We've also talked about how hormonal symptoms are often dismissed as "normal" when they're not, and how deeply our hormones influence everything from our energy levels and mood to our overall personality and daily functioning. Understanding these foundational elements empowers you to take charge of your hormonal health and better manage the symptoms that often accompany these phases of life.

In this chapter, we'll explore the significance of androgens, what happens when their levels are too high or too low, and how to harness your inner wonder woman by balancing these powerful hormones.

Testosterone is often labeled as the male hormone, but women produce it too, though in smaller quantities. In women, testosterone is essential for muscle strength, bone health, and sexual desire. It also plays a role in regulating mood and energy levels. Low testosterone can sap your energy, dull your drive, and turn even the simplest tasks into monumental efforts, while high levels can cause symptoms like acne, excessive hair growth, and irregular menstrual cycles. Interestingly enough, both high and low levels of testosterone can contribute to hair loss.

DHEA, or dehydroepiandrosterone, is another crucial androgen. It serves as a precursor to both estrogen and testosterone, meaning the body can convert it into either hormone as needed. DHEA is known for its anti-aging properties and its role in enhancing immune function, energy, and resilience to stress. Low levels of DHEA can lead to fatigue, reduced immune function, and a general sense of malaise, while high levels can contribute to symptoms similar to those of high testosterone.

The causes of androgen imbalances are varied. High levels of androgens can be due to genetic factors, insulin resistance, or adrenal gland disorders. Low levels can result from adrenal insufficiency, aging, chronic stress, or certain medical conditions. Identifying the root cause of the imbalance is crucial for effective treatment.

DHEA and testosterone play a unique and often underestimated role in how women navigate their inner and outer worlds. These hormones are not just about libido, bone density, or muscle mass; they are deeply intertwined with a woman's sense of self, drive, and courage. When androgen levels are balanced, you feel strong, assertive, and ready to tackle whatever comes your way. These hormones are the ones that give you the energy to power through your workouts, the confidence to speak up in meetings, and the drive to pursue your goals without hesitation. They help you set boundaries, take risks, and embrace your full, authentic self. In short, androgens are the hormones of action, helping you engage with life boldly and unapologetically.

One of the most fascinating aspects of androgens is their natural fluctuation during the menstrual cycle, particularly around ovulation. During this time, testosterone levels peak, boosting libido and enhancing the desire to connect with others, especially a partner. This surge in testosterone around mid-cycle is not just about physical attraction; it's a biological signal driving women to seek connection, intimacy, and assertiveness in their relationships. It's as if the body is primed for engagement—whether that's in the bedroom, in social settings, or in pursuing creative projects. This boost of testosterone can make you feel more confident, more attractive, and more in tune with your own desires, creating a window of opportunity to express yourself fully and authentically.

However, when androgen levels are low, the effects can be quite different—self-doubt creeps in, motivation wanes, and the drive to pursue goals or connect with others diminishes. Low levels can sap the joy out of things that once felt exciting or important, making even the smallest tasks feel overwhelming.

Low testosterone in women is more than just a physical deficit—it's a feeling of having no gas in the tank, a profound sense of listlessness that can drain motivation and zest for life. When testosterone levels are low, the drive to take action, tackle tasks, and engage with the world can diminish significantly, leaving you feeling stuck, unproductive, and disconnected from your usual sense of purpose. This isn't just about being tired; it's a deeper lack of motivation that can make even the simplest tasks feel insurmountable.

The emotional toll of this can be heavy, often leading to feelings of guilt and frustration, as you find yourself unable to accomplish what you set out to do. You might feel like you're constantly falling behind, blaming yourself for what feels like a lack of willpower, when in reality, it's your hormones that are sapping your energy and enthusiasm. Recognizing that these feelings may be tied to low hormones—and not a personal failing—can be the first step towards reclaiming your drive and rebalancing your inner strength.

In a world that often pressures women to be agreeable, accommodating, and "nice," balanced androgens provide the inner fire to push back, to say no, and to prioritize one's own needs without guilt. They are the hormones that help women break free from the constraints of traditional femininity, embracing a fuller, more dynamic expression of their whole selves. The role of androgens in women's health challenges the traditional view that women must always be soft, gentle, or deferential, instead celebrating the bold, adventurous, and unapologetically fierce aspects of femininity.

Having optimum androgen levels is about reclaiming the full spectrum of who you are. Whether it's the confidence to take on a new challenge, the energy to pursue a passion, or the desire to connect intimately with a partner, androgens play a pivotal role in empowering women to live authentically and powerfully. They remind us that feeling strong, capable, and alive isn't just about the absence of symptoms; it's about fully embracing the powerful, driven, and resilient woman within.

Understanding androgens and their role in your

health is key to harnessing your inner wonder woman, but it's equally important to view these hormones within the broader hormonal landscape. DHEA and testosterone don't operate in isolation—each hormone influences and is influenced by others. Progesterone can convert into testosterone, and testosterone can further convert into estrogen, creating a complex web of hormonal interactions. This interconnectedness means that supplementing with androgens, particularly testosterone, requires careful consideration and precise monitoring, as both too much and too little can have significant impacts. In fact, excessive testosterone can often be more disruptive than low levels, leading to a host of physical and emotional symptoms that can undermine well-being.

Recognizing the symptoms of imbalance and taking a holistic approach to address them empowers you to achieve optimal hormonal health. The goal is not just about boosting individual hormones, but about creating a harmonious balance that supports your vitality and strength. By understanding the interplay of androgens within your unique hormonal system, you can truly harness your inner power and enjoy a vibrant, energetic life.

CHAPTER 6

BECOME A THYROID DETECTIVE

Alright, now it's time to switch gears and talk about the thyroid, that small but mighty gland that's secretly running the show in your body. Nestled in your neck like a butterfly (it literally looks like a butterfly) on a mission, the thyroid regulates your metabolism, energy levels, mood, and even your heartbeat.

When it's doing its job, you probably don't even notice it. But when things go haywire? It's like your body's control center starts sending all the wrong signals, turning everything upside down. Let's dive in and uncover the mysteries of the thyroid, pinpoint when it's not functioning optimally, and explore how to get this vital gland back on the right path.

Think of your thyroid as the thermostat of your body. It produces key hormones—primarily thyroxine (T4) and triiodothyronine (T3)—that regulate how your body uses energy. These hormones influence nearly every cell in your body, dictating everything from how fast your heart beats to how efficiently you burn calories. T4 is like the backup fuel—it's the inactive form of thyroid hormone that must be converted into T3, the active form that actually revs up your metabolism. This conversion mostly takes place in the liver but also in other tissues like your gut and muscles, meaning that your thyroid function isn't just about the thyroid itself; it's a whole-body affair.

When your thyroid is working smoothly, it keeps your body humming along, finely tuned to your needs. But when this balance gets thrown off, it can lead to an underactive thyroid (hypothyroidism) or an overactive thyroid (hyperthyroidism), each bringing its own set of challenges and disruptions.

The commonly cited prevalence of hypothyroidism—around 4-5% of the general population—is likely an underestimation due to limitations in conventional testing and diagnostic criteria. Conventional medicine often relies primarily on TSH (thyroid-stimulating hormone) levels to diagnose hypothyroidism, which can miss many cases where symptoms are present but TSH remains within the so-called "normal" range. Thyroid health is about way more than just the gland itself; it's an intricate dance involving your brain, gut, liver, and immune system. Your pituitary gland, up in your brain, acts like the boss, sending TSH signals to the thyroid to pump out more T4 and T3. High TSH means the thyroid isn't keeping up—it's like your boss yelling, "Work harder!"

TSH is the test your doctor is usually referring to when they say, "We tested your thyroid, and it came back normal." The problem with this approach is that it often misses the mark due to what's known as a "faulty thermostat"—meaning the TSH measurement alone doesn't accurately reflect what's really happening with your thyroid. Time and again, I've worked with clients who have struggled with thyroid symptoms for years, only to be repeatedly told that their thyroid is "normal." It's not until we dig deeper and test their actual thyroid values—T4, T3, and thyroid antibodies—that the real story unfolds. More often than not, they do have a thyroid issue.

Holistic and functional medicine practitioners also consider the presence of symptoms that are often overlooked or dismissed by conventional standards. As a result, these experts suggest that the actual prevalence of hypothyroidism may be significantly higher, realistically ranging from 10-20% of the population. This is particularly true among women, older adults, and individuals with autoimmune conditions.

Many cases of subclinical hypothyroidism or atypical presentations are often undiagnosed or misdiagnosed, contributing to the growing belief among healthcare professionals that hypothyroidism is far more prevalent than traditionally recognized.

When your thyroid slows down, so does everything else: energy plummets, weight creeps up, and the world feels colder, both literally and figuratively. You might find yourself fighting fatigue, battling depression, struggling with weight gain, or feeling like you're wading through life in slow motion. For women, especially those entering midlife, these symptoms are often brushed off as just "getting older" or blamed on menopause. But let's be clear: feeling this way is not normal, and you deserve to feel vibrant at any age.

Hyperthyroidism, though much less common, flips the script, causing everything to speed up. Suddenly, your heart races, anxiety spikes, and you may lose weight rapidly without trying. It's like your body's internal engine is revving out of control, and without intervention, it can spiral into serious complications, particularly affecting your heart. Both hypo- and hyperthyroidism are influenced by autoimmune diseases, nutritional deficiencies, and stress, each acting like fuel on the fire of thyroid imbalance.

Autoimmune conditions like Hashimoto's and Graves' disease are often the culprits, with your immune system mistakenly attacking your thyroid, either slowing it down or putting it into overdrive. And then there's stress, that ever-present saboteur. Chronic stress floods your body with cortisol, a hormone that can interfere with the conversion of T4 to T3, throwing your thyroid off course even if the gland itself is technically healthy. It's like having the right ingredients but the wrong recipe—your thyroid is doing its best, but external factors are messing with the final product.

And let's not forget the nutritional side of the story. Your thyroid is a nutrient hog, needing specific vitamins and minerals like iodine, selenium, and zinc to function properly. Iodine is the raw material for thyroid hormone production, but both too much and too little can spell trouble—especially in the case of autoimmunity. Selenium is your gland's trusty bodyguard, protecting it from oxidative stress and aiding in the crucial conversion of T4 to T3. Zinc plays a dual role, supporting both thyroid hormone production and your immune system, making it a key player in overall thyroid health.

So how do you determine if a thyroid condition may be at the root of all your issues?

Start with your symptoms—they're your body's way of sending up the "something's off" signal. Fatigue, unexplained weight gain, anxiety, thinning hair, dry skin, mood swings—these are all clues that your thyroid might be out of sync. Don't let anyone brush you off with a "just stress" or "you're getting older" excuse; you deserve better.

Admittedly, this can be where things get a little tricky because many of the symptoms of low thyroid are common with other issues. For instance, is your thinning hair a thyroid issue, a low ferritin issue, a low or high testosterone issue, or an autoimmune condition? Are your fatigue and weight gain a cortisol issue or a thyroid issue? This is where laboratory data comes in. It can help you focus on what is actually going on vs. simply guessing.

That is why advocating for comprehensive testing is a must. A full thyroid panel—not just TSH—can provide the clues you need. Request tests for T4, free T3,and thyroid antibodies. These markers can reveal hidden issues that standard testing might miss, giving you a clearer picture of what's really going on with your thyroid. And remember, even if your levels fall within the "normal" range, that doesn't necessarily mean they're optimal for you. The goal is not just to fall within the numbers but to feel good.

If your thyroid is out of balance, there are steps you can take to help restore it. Diet and lifestyle are your foundation—ensuring you get the right nutrients, avoiding gluten, managing stress, and staying active can all support thyroid health. If needed, thyroid hormone replacement therapy is an option, but it's not one-size-fits-all. Some people do well on synthetic T4 alone, while others need a combination of T4 and T3, or even natural desiccated thyroid, which provides both hormones in their bio-identical forms.

Given the complexity of thyroid conditions, it's crucial to consider the underlying causes, particularly autoimmunity. At least 80% of low thyroid cases are due to an autoimmune attack on the thyroid, often Hashimoto's thyroiditis, even if standard tests don't always show clear autoimmune markers. This means that the immune system mistakenly targets the thyroid gland, causing it to underperform over time. There are many potential targets for autoimmunity on the thyroid, including thyroid peroxidase (TPO) and thyroglobulin, which are essential proteins involved in thyroid hormone production. These autoimmune attacks can quietly cause significant damage long before thyroid hormone levels fall out of the "normal" range, leading to symptoms like fatigue, weight gain, and brain fog.

It's important to remember that while there are only a handful of tests available to detect thyroid autoimmunity, these tests don't tell the whole story. In reality, there are thousands of different potential targets for autoimmune attacks on the thyroid, most of which we simply don't have tests for yet. So, if your antibody tests come back normal, it doesn't necessarily mean your thyroid isn't under attack.

One of the most telling signs of an autoimmune issue, even when antibody tests are negative, is a low Total T4 level. Total T4 measures the overall amount of thyroid hormone your body is producing. If this number is consistently low or shows significant fluctuations across multiple tests, it's a strong indicator that something isn't right behind the scenes, suggesting that an autoimmune process may still be at play.

For those with thyroid conditions, going gluten-free is not just a trendy option to make your friends roll their eyes; it's a critical part of managing and mitigating autoimmunity. Gluten, a protein found in wheat, barley, rye, and other grains can mimic thyroid tissue on a molecular level due to a process called molecular mimicry.

This means that when your body's immune system reacts to gluten, it can mistakenly attack the thyroid as well, fueling the autoimmune response and worsening thyroid dysfunction. By eliminating gluten, you reduce one of the most common triggers that can perpetuate this mistaken identity, helping to calm the immune system and protect thyroid function. For anyone with thyroid imbalances, especially those suspected of being autoimmune in nature, going gluten-free is the best tip you'll ever get.

This is not just a half-hearted suggestion either. If you have an underactive thyroid there is a 80% chance that it is autoimmune related. Individuals with autoimmune attacks on their thyroid have a 10x greater chance of developing thyroid cancer than the general population. Any cyst or nodule needs to be monitored closer with frequent ultrasounds. Going gluten-free calms the autoimmune attack, reducing this risk. In addition you can apply a topical glutathione cream or castor oil to help shrink any nodules or cysts.

Ultimately, your thyroid health is about understanding your body's signals, getting the right information, and making informed choices that support you. Being a thyroid detective means listening to your body, connecting the dots, and advocating for the care you deserve. If your doctor has repeatedly told you that your thyroid is "normal" but you still feel off, it's time to get a second opinion—or take matters into your own hands. You don't have to be at the mercy of a medical system that might overlook the nuances of thyroid health. At-home tests are available, allowing you to bypass the frustration of trying to convince a doctor and instead get the answers you need.

By becoming your own thyroid detective, you can actively listen to your body, understand what's really going on, and access the right tests to get the full picture. Whether you're managing symptoms of an underactive or overactive thyroid or just want to ensure your thyroid is functioning at its best, taking a proactive approach can significantly improve your quality of life.

CHAPTER 7

LET'S TALK ABOUT SEX BABY

Sexual health is a big part of overall well-being, yet it often gets pushed aside when hormones are out of balance. When you're grappling with thyroid issues, dysregulated cortisol, or other hormonal imbalances, the idea of intimacy can feel exhausting. Fatigue, mood swings, and body aches can make sex seem more like a chore than something to enjoy.

Add to that the brain fog and anxiety that often accompany hormonal fluctuations, and it's easy to see how sex falls to the bottom of the priority list. However, sexual health is not just about pleasure (though that's incredibly important); regular orgasms bring numerous health benefits, such as boosting mood, easing pain, improving sleep, and deepening your emotional connection with your partner.

Hormonal imbalances, particularly during menopause, are notorious for turning the heat way down on your libido. As estrogen levels drop, vaginal dryness can make sex uncomfortable or even painful, leading many women to avoid intimacy altogether. The natural decline in progesterone and dysregulated cortisol levels can trigger anxiety, irritability, and sleeplessness, making it hard to even consider intimacy. Menopause can feel like a particularly rough patch when it comes to sex, as hot flashes, night sweats, and weight gain leave you feeling anything but sexy. All of these changes can affect your confidence and overall sense of well-being, and it can become challenging to embrace your body and its evolving needs.

Intimacy during menopause doesn't have to be an uphill battle. Staying connected—whether through touch, laughter, or simply being present—helps maintain intimacy. Using lubricants designed to address vaginal dryness can make intimacy more comfortable. If needed, consult your doctor about topical treatments like estriol cream, a safe option that doesn't contribute to estrogen dominance but alleviates discomfort. Choosing hormone-friendly lubricants free of endocrine disruptors can also make a world of difference; we've linked some recommended products in the book's reference section.

For men, erectile dysfunction (ED) often signals

that testosterone levels have been low for a while. It's more than just a performance issue; it impacts confidence, connection, and overall well-being. When ED appears, it's usually a wake-up call to examine lifestyle factors such as stress, diet, and exercise. Regular physical activity, a balanced diet, and stress management can help support male hormone health, but if symptoms persist, seeking professional help is crucial.

The good news is that many herbal remedies can help enhance libido and address hormonal imbalances, which we will cover in the next chapter. Remember, it's not just about hormone levels; mindset and connection play huge roles. When you're exhausted, stressed, or simply not feeling great about yourself, intimacy can feel like just another to-do list item.

When libido takes a dip, it's time to rekindle the spark by focusing on sensation and pleasure rather than the end goal. Communication is key—share your desires, boundaries, and any discomforts with your partner. Taking breaks, teasing, and experimenting with positions can make intimacy more enjoyable and less stressful. For menopausal women, positions like modified missionary (with a pillow under the hips), woman-on-top for control, and side-by-side for intimacy can help make sex more comfortable. Oral sex and clitoral stimulation can also lead to more intense orgasms, providing a sense of satisfaction and closeness with your partner.

Breathing exercises can also enhance sexual pleasure by reducing stress, increasing oxygenation, and improving focus. Here are a few exercises to try:

1. Diaphragmatic Breathing: Inhale deeply through your nose, allowing your belly to rise as you fill your lungs with air. Exhale slowly through your mouth, letting your belly fall. Repeat this for a few minutes to relax your body and calm your mind.

2. 4-7-8 Breathing: Inhale through your nose for a count of 4. Hold your breath for a count of 7. Then, exhale through your mouth for a count of 8. This exercise helps to reduce anxiety and promotes relaxation, setting the stage for a more connected experience.

3. Alternate Nostril Breathing: Close one nostril with your finger and inhale through the other. Switch and exhale through the opposite nostril. Alternate between nostrils to help balance your nervous system and increase relaxation.

4. Box Breathing: Inhale through your nose for a

count of 4, hold your breath for a count of 4, exhale for a count of 4, and hold again for a count of 4. Repeat this process to center your mind and increase blood flow to your body.

Incorporating these breathing exercises into your routine helps you stay present, relax, and enhance the sensory experience during intimacy. They can also improve orgasmic potential by increasing oxygenation and circulation throughout the body.

Beyond physical techniques, intimacy can be further deepened by focusing on activities that build trust, communication, and connection. For example, engaging in sensual massages can help you and your partner connect physically and emotionally. Intimate yoga sessions with partner poses allow for shared experiences that build both physical and emotional flexibility. Simple acts like maintaining eye contact during touch or movement can also significantly enhance intimacy, making both partners feel more present and connected.

Ultimately, enhancing your sexual health involves a multi-faceted approach. It's about balancing hormones, reducing stress, exploring new activities, and maintaining open communication with your partner. Embrace where you are, address any hormonal roadblocks, and make pleasure a priority—it's good for your hormones, your heart, and your happiness. Check out the resources at the back of this book for additional tips, techniques, and products to help you reignite your passion and connection.

CHAPTER 8

MYTHS AND MISCONCEPTIONS OF MEN'S HORMONE HEALTH

While this book has focused primarily on women's hormonal health, it's equally important to recognize that men face their own set of challenges when it comes to hormones. The modern world, with its high levels of stress, environmental toxins, poor diet, and sedentary lifestyles, has led to a silent epidemic of hormonal imbalances in men, most notably low testosterone.

Testosterone is often thought of as the quintessential male hormone, crucial not only for libido and muscle mass but also for energy, mood, and overall vitality. Yet, many men today are experiencing a dramatic decline in testosterone levels, sometimes even in their 20s and 30s, which is both concerning and indicative of broader health issues.

Low testosterone isn't just about feeling tired

or having a low sex drive; it's a condition that affects nearly every aspect of a man's physical and mental health. Unfortunately, erectile dysfunction is often the only symptom that gets attention from healthcare providers, leading to a focus on quick fixes rather than addressing the broader impact of low testosterone on a man's life. This narrow approach is a disservice to men, as low testosterone can also manifest as fatigue, depression, anxiety, loss of drive, decreased ambition, and an overall sense of listlessness.

These symptoms can severely impact a man's quality of life, making him feel like he's lost his edge or zest for living. There is also a strong correlation between low testosterone, increased belly fat, and depression, creating a vicious cycle in which low testosterone contributes to weight gain, which then further lowers testosterone levels, compounding feelings of hopelessness and low self-esteem.

Another factor to consider is andropause, often referred to as the male equivalent of menopause, where testosterone levels decline naturally with age. This gradual decline can lead to many of the same symptoms experienced by women during menopause, including mood swings, irritability, and a loss of mental clarity. However, because the decline is often slower and less abrupt than in women, it often goes unrecognized and untreated, leaving men struggling without answers.

Estrogen dominance is another underrecognized issue for men. It occurs when the balance between progesterone and estrogen shifts unfavorably, either due to increased estrogen levels or insufficient progesterone. Symptoms of estrogen dominance in men can include weight gain, especially around the chest and belly, low libido, erectile dysfunction, mood swings, and the development of gynecomastia (enlarged breast tissue). This imbalance is frequently compounded by an overactive aromatase enzyme, which converts testosterone into estrogen at an accelerated rate. This enzyme is particularly busy in men with extra body fat or insulin resistance, or those who enjoy a few too many beers, creating a double whammy of low testosterone and high estrogen.

Add to this the constant exposure to endocrine disruptors—chemicals found in plastics, pesticides, and industrial materials—and you've got a recipe for hormonal chaos. These chemicals act like rogue agents in the body, mimicking or blocking hormones and throwing off internal balance. Men working in manufacturing, automotive repair, or construction are especially at risk, regularly encountering substances like BPA (found in plastics), phthalates, and heavy metals like lead. All of these disrupt testosterone production, paving the way for hormonal imbalances that can turn their body's inner workings upside down.

Another crucial hormone often overlooked in men is progesterone. Known as the "mother hormone," progesterone plays a foundational role in the body's hormonal cascade, including the production of testosterone. Progesterone has protective effects against estrogen dominance and helps to balance the effects of excess estrogen by acting as a natural aromatase inhibitor, thereby reducing the conversion of testosterone into estrogen. Unfortunately, progesterone levels can also be low in men, especially as they age or experience chronic stress. Supporting progesterone levels can have a profound impact on balancing overall hormonal health, yet it's rarely considered in standard treatment protocols for men.

So, what's a guy to do when testosterone is tanking, and hormones are in disarray? The knee-jerk response is often testosterone replacement therapy (TRT), but let's not be too hasty. While TRT can boost testosterone levels quickly, it can also suppress your body's natural production, leading to dependence on external testosterone and even affecting fertility. It's like hitting the override button on your body's control panel—effective in the short term but potentially problematic down the road.

Instead of jumping straight to TRT, I often prefer a more nuanced approach that supports the body's own hormone production. Glandulars, for instance, can provide the necessary raw materials to stimulate the body's natural hormone-making systems. Adrenal, testicular, and pituitary glandulars help support the endocrine system by providing bioavailable nutrients that bolster the body's natural hormone production processes. In addition, progesterone and DHEA are invaluable tools in the male hormonal toolkit. Both of these hormones are precursors to testosterone, meaning they can naturally support the body's ability to produce testosterone without the disruptive side effects of direct testosterone replacement.

The key to effective hormone management in men is to address the root causes of imbalance rather than simply treating symptoms. This means supporting the body's natural hormonal pathways, addressing lifestyle factors that contribute to hormonal disruption, and using targeted supplements to assist where needed. By taking a holistic approach, it's possible to achieve optimal hormonal health without compromising long-term well-being or fertility.

Men's hormonal health is often an afterthought in the broader conversation about wellness, but it deserves just as much attention and care. Understanding the complexities of testosterone, estrogen, progesterone, and DHEA can empower men to make informed decisions about their health and take control of their hormonal balance. By focusing on natural, supportive approaches rather than quick fixes, we can help men feel their best at any age.

CHAPTER 9

HORMONE HAVOC, MEET SUPPLEMENT SOLUTIONS

Navigating hormonal imbalances can feel overwhelming, but supplements can be key allies in restoring balance. From easing PMS to managing perimenopause, the right supplements can make a significant impact on daily well-being. In this chapter, we'll explore the most effective supplements for hormone health—how they work, why they work, and how to use them wisely. We'll also discuss bio-identical hormones for those needing a more customized approach. If you're ready to tackle mood swings, irregular cycles, or hot flashes, let's dive in!

Supplements for Overall Hormone Balance

Calcium D-glucarate acts as a detoxifier, supporting the liver in clearing out excess estrogen. This supplement is especially helpful for those dealing with estrogen dominance and can aid in reducing PMS symptoms, heavy periods, and mood swings by preventing reabsorption of processed estrogen.

Sulforaphane, found in cruciferous vegetables like broccoli, enhances the liver's detox pathways, clearing excess hormones and toxins. Its anti-inflammatory properties make it particularly valuable for women dealing with estrogen dominance or irregular cycles.

DIM (Diindolylmethane), also found in cruciferous vegetables like broccoli and kale, promotes the conversion of estrogen into "good" metabolites, reducing symptoms like weight gain, mood swings, and hormonal acne. It's especially useful for those with conditions like polycystic ovary syndrome (PCOS).

Vitex (Chaste Tree Berry) supports the pituitary gland, helping to regulate estrogen and progesterone levels. This ancient remedy is particularly beneficial for women experiencing PMS, irregular cycles, or perimenopause, offering a natural way to rebalance hormone levels.

Wild Yam: Contains diosgenin, a compound that can mimic progesterone in the body, helping to balance hormones and potentially alleviate symptoms of PMS and menopause.

GoldenRoot™, my personal favorite and proprietary formulation, is crafted in small batches in a Health Canada-approved laboratory. This organic turmeric blend includes ginger, black pepper, oregano, and lavender, designed to support hormone balance, immune health, and overall wellness. It reduces inflammation, alleviates pain, and supports brain and gut health, making it beneficial for managing anxiety, stress, and concussion-related symptoms. GoldenRoot™ is gluten-free, vegan, and highly absorbable. For more information, visit GoldenRoot™ (https://manoticknaturalmarket.com/products/golden-root)

Combination products often blend DIM, calcium D-glucarate, vitex, sulforaphane and other herbs for comprehensive hormone support, making it easier to address multiple imbalances at once.

Supplements for Thyroid Support

When your thyroid is out of balance, it can throw off your entire system. Here's how to support it:

Selenium is crucial for converting inactive T4 into the active T3 hormone. It also acts as an antioxidant, protecting the thyroid from oxidative stress and inflammation. By neutralizing harmful by-products like hydrogen peroxide, selenium helps maintain a smoothly functioning thyroid and prevents autoimmune attacks on the gland.

Vitamin A enhances hormone receptor sensitivity, ensuring hormones like thyroid hormones can bind effectively and trigger the correct cellular responses. It also aids in converting T4 to T3, promoting balanced energy levels and overall hormonal health.

Iodine is necessary for thyroid hormone production. However, it's a mineral that requires careful balancing—both deficiency and excess can disrupt thyroid function. While some experts advocate for iodine supplementation, others caution against it, particularly in those with autoimmune thyroid conditions like Hashimoto's thyroiditis. Excess iodine can increase hydrogen peroxide production, leading to oxidative damage and inflammation. The key is balancing iodine with other nutrients, such as selenium and glutathione, which neutralize its potential negative effects. Therefore, iodine supplementation should always be undertaken under the guidance of a healthcare professional.

Supplements to Support the Adrenals

Your adrenal glands are key players in hormone balance, especially when dealing with chronic stress. Proper adrenal support can prevent hormonal imbalances from spiraling out of control:

Phosphatidylserine helps regulate the body's stress response by lowering elevated cortisol levels. It supports brain function, improves mood, and aids recovery from prolonged stress.

Adaptogenic herbs like ashwagandha and rhodiola modulate cortisol, reduce anxiety, and boost overall stress resilience. If combined with B vitamins, they provide comprehensive support for the adrenals, enhancing the body's ability to manage daily stressors.

Glandular Supplements

Glandular supplements provide targeted support for specific glands, such as the ovaries, thyroid, and adrenals. They contain extracts from animal glands, supplying nutrients and growth factors that nourish and support the body's glandular systems:

- Thyroid glandulars help stimulate hormone production, particularly beneficial for those with a sluggish thyroid.
- Ovarian glandulars for women balance reproductive hormones, especially during perimenopause.
- Testicular glandulars for men support testosterone production and overall reproductive health.
- Adrenal glandulars support natural cortisol

production, aiding in stress resilience.

Glandulars can nudge the body's glands to function more efficiently, but effectiveness hinges on sourcing high-quality, clean products free of harmful additives.

Additional supplements to Support HRT or Birth Control Pill Use

For those on hormone replacement therapy or birth control pills, certain supplements help counteract nutrient depletions caused by these medications:

Magnesium is a multitasker, essential for managing stress, supporting sleep, and aiding hormone metabolism. Magnesium glycinate or bisglycinate are the best forms for hormonal support due to their high absorbability and gentle effects on the digestive system. These forms also promote relaxation, making them particularly effective for stress and insomnia.

B Vitamins play a key role in adrenal support, energy production, and neurotransmitter balance. B5 aids in managing stress by supporting adrenal function, while B6 is crucial for neurotransmitter synthesis and mood regulation. B12 and folate support energy production and stress resilience. Choosing bioavailable forms, like methylfolate and methylcobalamin, ensures optimal absorption, especially for those with genetic or gut health issues.

Additional Supportive Nutrients

Here are some additional nutrients that have been studied for hormone balancing as well as mood and libido enhancers. You will find many of these herbs in combination products.

Phytoestrogens

1. Black Cohosh: Alleviates hot flashes, vaginal dryness, and low libido.

2. Red Clover: May improve estrogen levels and sexual function.

3. Dong Quai: Traditional Chinese herb for hormonal balance and libido.

4. Ginseng: Enhances energy, vitality, and sexual desire.

Aphrodisiacs

1. Maca: Peruvian plant known for its libido-boosting properties.

2. Ashwagandha: Reduces stress, improves energy, and enhances sexual function.

3. Damiana: Traditional Mexican herb for female

libido and arousal.

4. Yohimbe: Stimulates blood flow, improving sexual sensation.

Mood Enhancers

1. St. John's Wort: Mild antidepressant that improves mood and libido.
2. 5HTP: A precursor to serotonin, it can positively impact low mood.
3. Passionflower: Reduces anxiety, promoting relaxation and intimacy.
4. Rosemary: Enhances circulation, improving sensory experience.

Libido Enhancers

1. Ginseng: Boosts energy, vitality, and sexual desire.
2. Maca: Enhances libido with its natural properties.
3. Ashwagandha: Reduces stress and supports sexual function.
4. Tribulus Terrestris: Increases testosterone levels and libido.
5. Damiana: Enhances male libido and arousal.

6. Horny Goat Weed (Epimedium): Improves blood flow and erectile function.
7. Yohimbe: Stimulates blood flow, supporting erectile function.

Erectile Function Support

1. L-Arginine: Improves blood flow and nitric oxide production.
2. Ginkgo Biloba: Enhances blood flow to the genitals.
3. Muira Puama: Brazilian herb for better erectile function and libido.
4. Saw Palmetto: May alleviate testosterone-related symptoms to improve libido.
5. Tongkat Ali (Eurycoma Longifolia): Enhances testosterone and libido.
6. My Goldenroot™: A blend of turmeric, ginger, oregano, black pepper, and lavender to boost energy, reduce inflammation, and support blood flow.

Testosterone Support

1. D-Aspartic Acid (DAA): An amino acid that supports testosterone production.
2. Fenugreek: Naturally increases testosterone

levels and libido.

3. Mucuna Pruriens: Boosts dopamine and testosterone levels

4. Zinc: Zinc is crucial for testosterone production, particularly in men, where it supports normal levels and overall reproductive health. In women, zinc can aid in reducing symptoms of excess testosterone by balancing overall hormone levels.

When choosing supplements, focus on your symptoms and areas where you need the most support, whether it's PMS, irregular cycles, or thyroid issues. Consulting a healthcare provider knowledgeable in hormonal health can help tailor your approach. Always opt for high-quality supplements from reputable brands to ensure you're getting what your body needs without harmful additives. Start with the recommended dose, monitor how your body responds, and adjust as necessary. Remember, more is not always better; the goal is to find the right balance that works for you.

By understanding these supplements and incorporating them thoughtfully into your routine, you can take control of your hormonal health and find the balance your body craves.

BioIdentical Hormones

When it comes to bioidentical hormone replacement therapy (BHRT), it's a hot topic, and for a good reason. All my clients ask me about it, and while I'm a big fan, there's always a "but" to consider. BHRT can be life-changing, providing a more personalized approach to managing hormonal imbalances. However, it requires a thoughtful and careful strategy.

Bioidentical hormone therapy comes in various forms: patches, creams, oral tablets, sprays, and pellets, each with its benefits and drawbacks. Patches deliver a steady hormone dose, but some people find them irritating to the skin. Oral options, like Prometrium, are convenient but involve liver processing and contain peanut oil, so they're not suitable for those with allergies. Pellets, inserted under the skin, provide long-term release but aren't easily adjusted once in place, complicating dose fine-tuning or troubleshooting reactions. Creams and sprays bypass the liver, allowing smoother absorption and quick dosage adjustments. Sprays, in particular, dry quickly without leaving a residue, offering a discreet application method. It's for these reasons that creams and sprays are my preferred modes of hormone replacement therapy.

One of the biggest misconceptions is that more hormones mean better results. This "more is better" mentality can lead to complications, especially if therapy is approached without understanding the delicate balance of our body's hormone system. Overloading on hormones can overwhelm the liver, particularly if it's already dealing with other stressors like medications, alcohol, or chronic illness. This strain can lead to improper clearance of hormones, causing them to be reabsorbed into the bloodstream and worsening symptoms. That's why finding the right dose and combination is crucial, and why it's important to work closely with a knowledgeable healthcare provider.

Proper testing is the backbone of effective BHRT. Too often, only blood tests are used to gauge hormone levels, but these only provide a limited snapshot. They don't necessarily reflect the hormones that are actively available to your cells. This is where saliva testing becomes a game-changer, as it measures the hormones that your cells can actually use, especially important when monitoring sex hormones and cortisol levels. With BHRT, regular testing every three months is a must to ensure hormone levels stay within an optimal range and to adjust dosages as needed. Hormone levels can fluctuate rapidly due to stress, viral infections, liver function, or medications like steroids. Frequent monitoring keeps these levels in check, helping you avoid both under- and over-replacement.

Understanding hormone interaction is another key element often overlooked in BHRT. Hormones don't operate in isolation; they convert into each other depending on various factors in the body. For example, DHEA can turn into testosterone or estrogen based on the body's needs, a process influenced by enzymes like aromatase. Factors such as inflammation, insulin resistance, or obesity can boost aromatase activity, resulting in higher estrogen levels. Supplementing hormones without taking these interactions into account can quickly lead to imbalance. This is why precision in both testing and treatment is essential for successful BHRT.

Then there's the temptation of over-the-counter hormone products like DHEA, progesterone creams, and estriol. While these options can seem convenient, using them without proper guidance can disrupt your hormone balance. For example, DHEA dosing is specific—typically 5 to 10 mg for women, but much more for men. I've seen cases where women unknowingly took doses meant for men, resulting in elevated testosterone or estrogen levels, making their symptoms worse. Similarly, progesterone, while beneficial, can convert into other hormones like cortisol, testosterone, or estrogen, depending on what the body needs. Too high of a dose can throw everything out of balance, leading to increased cortisol and amplifying stress.

On a more positive note, estriol cream offers a gentle and effective solution for vaginal dryness and discomfort. Estriol, a weaker form of estrogen, remains mostly localized, working to improve vaginal tissues without raising overall estrogen levels. This makes it an excellent option for those who are concerned about estrogen dominance but need relief from symptoms like dryness or discomfort during intimacy. Estriol can enhance vaginal elasticity and natural lubrication, promoting comfort and a sense of well-being.

Ultimately, the goal with hormone therapy should always be to use the minimum effective dose to achieve the desired results. Unfortunately, many women are prescribed a cocktail of hormones—estrogen, progesterone, testosterone, and DHEA—without proper evaluation of their specific needs. This approach often creates a hormonal storm that's hard to manage. Instead, BHRT should be tailored, monitored, and adjusted based on regular testing and the individual's unique hormonal ecosystem.

In addition to BHRT, supplements can be invaluable in supporting hormone balance. Compounds like DIM, calcium D-glucarate, and sulforaphane help regulate the enzymes involved in hormone metabolism, offering a way to fine-tune the body's hormonal environment without resorting to high doses of hormone supplementation.

Bioidentical hormones mimic the exact chemical structure of the hormones naturally produced by the body, making them more easily absorbed and utilized. They can address a wide range of symptoms, including hot flashes, night sweats, mood swings, and sleep disturbances. However, using BHRT successfully involves not just taking hormones but understanding the broader picture.

Choosing BHRT should be a carefully considered decision, one that involves proper testing, ongoing monitoring, and a clear understanding of how each hormone interacts with the others. With the right guidance and approach, bio-identical hormones can be a powerful tool in managing hormonal health, but they must be used with respect for the delicate hormonal ecosystem that governs your body.

CHAPTER 10

TAKING CHARGE OF YOUR HORMONAL HEALTH

As we've journeyed through this book, we've delved into the complex and often misunderstood world of hormones. We've explored the ins and outs of these tiny but mighty chemical messengers, understanding how they influence everything from your mood and energy to metabolism and overall vitality. You've learned the secrets of estrogen, progesterone, testosterone, cortisol, thyroid hormones, and more.

The big takeaway? You are not at the mercy of your hormones—you're in the driver's seat, and with the right tools, you can take control of your health and reclaim your spark at any age.

From PMS to perimenopause, andropause, thyroid disorders, and adrenal fatigue, these conditions are signals from your body that something is out of balance. Hormonal health is not just about treating symptoms but understanding the root causes—whether it's stress, diet, environmental toxins, or underlying autoimmune conditions—

and addressing them holistically.

Hormonal imbalances can significantly impact mental health, drive, ambition, and overall quality of life, but they are often brushed aside or attributed to aging, work stress, or other nonspecific causes.

The first step in addressing any hormonal imbalance is proper testing. Start by getting comprehensive blood work that includes vitamin D (hormone D) and ferritin, as low ferritin can mimic many of the symptoms associated with hormonal imbalances, such as fatigue, brain fog, and mood swings.

For thyroid health, ensure you get a full thyroid panel that includes TSH, Total T4, free T3, and thyroid antibodies (TPOAb and TgAb). If your doctor is unwilling or unable to order these tests, home testing kits are available and can be a great alternative for getting the information you need. Remember, not all tests provide the full picture—standard blood tests often fall short when it comes to accurately measuring hormones, especially those delivered through topical creams or gels. It's vital to seek comprehensive testing that provides a true snapshot of what's going on in your body.

Finding a provider who understands hormonal

health is essential. Look for someone who can perform salivary hormone and adrenal profiles and knows how to interpret the results holistically—not just looking at the individual hormones, but understanding the full pattern, including the interplay between thyroid numbers and adrenal health. Saliva testing is particularly useful for measuring active hormone levels, especially if you're already on hormone replacement therapy, as it reflects the hormones available to your tissues rather than just circulating levels in the blood. Understanding the interaction between cortisol, estrogen, progesterone, testosterone, and thyroid hormones is crucial, as these hormones do not act independently; they interact like pieces of a complex puzzle, influencing each other in various ways.

Wherever possible, start with diet, lifestyle changes, and supplements before opting for hormone replacement. Reducing stress, getting quality sleep, exercising according to your cycle, and eating a balanced diet rich in whole foods can make a profound difference in your hormonal health. Supplements such as magnesium, B vitamins, adaptogenic herbs, and targeted glandulars can support your body's natural hormonal pathways, often without the need for additional hormone replacement. Check out the references, resources, and checklists we've added to the back of the book for specific guidance on dietary strategies, recommended supplements, and lifestyle changes tailored to your symptoms. These tools will help you craft a personalized approach that addresses your unique needs.

If hormone replacement is necessary, use the lowest effective dose to achieve the desired results, and always retest every three months until your symptoms and data are stable. After that, retest every six months or whenever symptoms change or new ones appear. Hormone therapy is not a "set it and forget it" solution; it requires careful monitoring and adjustments as your body's needs change. Bio-identical hormones can be a game-changer, but only when used thoughtfully and with a full understanding of the delicate balance between hormones.

Educate the women in your life—your daughters, nieces, sisters, and friends—about the signs of hormonal imbalance. The earlier these issues are identified and corrected, the better their long-term health will be. For those in their 20s and 30s, protecting adrenal health is key; don't burn yourself out with relentless stress and overwork. Recognize the early signs of imbalance and take action.

If you're in your 40s and 50s, remember that you don't have to suffer through perimenopause or menopause. There are effective strategies to manage your symptoms, from lifestyle changes to bio-identical hormone replacement when needed. And if you're in your late 50s and beyond, know that your hormones still matter. Supporting your adrenals, thyroid, and addressing ongoing conditions like PCOS or estrogen dominance is crucial to maintaining your health and quality of life. Persistent menopausal symptoms like hot flashes and night sweats later in life are not normal and deserve attention.

If you have a thyroid condition, especially one with autoimmune origins, going gluten-free is a must. The immune system's attack on the thyroid can extend to other tissues over time, leading to additional autoimmune diagnoses. Eliminating gluten is a simple but powerful step that can reduce immune activation and protect your thyroid from further damage. For those with persistent symptoms, diet alone may not be enough; consider additional strategies such as supplementation, glandular support, stress management, and avoiding endocrine disruptors to further support thyroid function.

Don't waste energy trying to convince doctors, friends, or family who aren't open to these less conventional approaches. Physicians are highly trained, dedicated professionals, but many work within the confines of traditional medical training, which often overlooks the nuanced needs of hormonal health. Instead, seek out practitioners who are well-versed in functional and integrative medicine—those who understand the whole-body approach to hormonal balance. The same goes for friends and family; everyone's journey is different, and not everyone will be ready to embrace new information or make changes.

Your next steps should be clear: begin by gathering the data you need with the right testing, seek knowledgeable providers, and start with foundational changes before moving on to more intensive interventions like hormone replacement therapy. If HRT is required, opt for bio-identical hormones and use the least amount necessary to restore balance. Regularly retest and adjust as needed, staying attuned to how your body responds.

Above all, know that hormonal health is not just about surviving—it's about thriving. Hormones influence every facet of who you are, from your energy and mood to your motivation and resilience. Taking charge of your hormonal health is one of the most empowering steps you can take for your overall well-being. Equip yourself with the knowledge, tools, and support you need to navigate this journey confidently, and remember: you deserve to feel vibrant and in control of your health at every stage of life. For more guidance, check out the resources at the back of the book to continue your path to balanced hormones and a better quality of life.

Hormonal health is an ongoing journey—embrace it, own it, and make it yours.

REFERENCES AND TOOLS

In this section, you'll find a comprehensive list of tools, references, and guides to help you on your journey toward hormonal health and overall well-being. Each section offers insights, practical tips, and resources to support a healthier lifestyle.

1. Resources For weight Loss and Context Eating
2. Recipes: Darpan's Hormone Balancing Menu Plan
3. Hormone Imbalance Symptom Checklist
4. Endocrine Disruptor Product Checklist
5. Common Endocrine Disruptors Chemical/ Ingredient Names
6. Information on Comprehensive Salivary Hormone Testing and Blood- Spot Full Thyroid Panel Testing
7. Links to Supplement Protocols and Trusted Brands

Resources for Weight Loss and Context Eating

For weight loss and a balanced eating approach that eliminates all or nothing approaches learn how to context eat with "The Context Eating Method."

Go to https://contexteatingmethod.com for more information

Access your FREE evaluation that will help you get to the root of your cravings and overeating https://contexteatingmethod.com/guide-1

Enroll in our 12 week self-study course to ditch dieting for good https://contexteatingmethod.com/12weekselfstudyorderform

Pick up The Context Eating Method for Women book or leave a review on Amazon

Canadian Customers
https://www.amazon.ca/Context-Eating-Method-Women-Wine-Filled/dp/1738822710

US Customers
https://www.amazon.com/-/he/Darpan-Ahluwalia/dp/1738822710

Pick up The Context Eating Method for Women book or leave a review on Audible https://us.amazon.com/Context-Eating-Method-Women-Wine-Filled/dp/B0C4Z7HD5V

Darpan's Hormone Balancing Menu Plan

- Day 1 -

- Breakfast: GF Oatmeal with almond butter (complex carbs, potassium, and healthy fats)

- Lunch: Grilled salmon with avocado salad topped with My GoldenrootTM (omega-3 fatty acids and vitamin E)

- Dinner: Beef, spinach and mushroom stir-fry with garlic and ginger (folate, antioxidants, and aphrodisiac properties)

- Snack: Dark chocolate-covered strawberries (flavonoids and phenylethylamine)

- Day 2 -

- Breakfast: Scrambled eggs with spinach and GF toast (protein, iron, and complex carbs)

- Lunch: Turkey and avocado wrap with mixed greens (protein, healthy fats, and fiber)

- Dinner: Grilled shrimp with sweet potato and steamed broccoli topped with My GoldenrootTM (vitamin B12, complex carbs, and antioxidants)

- Snack: Pineapple, protein, and coconut milk smoothie (vitamin C and medium-chain triglycerides)

- Day 3 -

- Breakfast: Greek yogurt with berries and raw honey 1 tsp of My GoldenrootTM (protein, calcium, and antioxidants)

- Lunch: Grilled chicken breast with quinoa and roasted cruciferous vegetables (protein, complex carbs, and fiber)

- Dinner: Beef and mushroom stew with red wine (iron, zinc, and antioxidants)

- Snack: Apple slices with almond butter (fiber, healthy fats, and antioxidants)

- Day 4 -

- Breakfast: Smoothie bowl with spinach, banana, and chia seeds and 1 tsp My GoldenrootTM (folate, potassium, and omega-3 fatty acids)

- Lunch: Turkey meatball sub with marinara sauce and GF bread (protein, complex carbs, and lycopene)

- Dinner: Grilled salmon with asparagus, lemon and parmesan cheese (Omegas, vitamin C, folate, and calcium)

- Snack: Dark chocolate-dipped apricots (flavonoids and phenylethylamine)

- Day 5 -

- Breakfast: Avocado (GF) toast with scrambled eggs and cherry tomatoes (healthy fats, protein, and lycopene)

- Lunch: Grilled chicken Caesar salad added 1/2 tsp of My GoldenrootTM (protein, complex carbs, and vitamin K)

- Dinner: Baked salmon with roasted Brussels sprouts and sweet potato (omega-3 fatty acids, vitamin C, and complex carbs)

- Snack: Coconut water with lime and mint (electrolytes and antioxidants)

- Day 6 -

- Breakfast: Omelette with mushrooms, spinach, and feta cheese (protein, folate, and calcium)

- Lunch: Grilled beef burger patty with avocado and sweet potato fries (protein, healthy fats, and complex carbs)

- Dinner: Shrimp and cruciferous vegetable skewers with quinoa topped with garlic olive oil and My GoldenrootTM (protein, complex carbs, and fiber)

- Snack: Watermelon and feta salad (vitamin C,

lycopene, and calcium)

- Day 7 -

- Breakfast: Scrambled eggs, GF waffles with strawberries and real whipped cream (complex carbs, vitamin C, and antioxidants)

- Lunch: Chicken and quinoa bowl with roasted cruciferous vegetables (protein, complex carbs, and fiber)

- Dinner: Grilled steak with roasted asparagus and garlic mashed potatoes (iron, vitamin C, and complex carbs)

- Snack: Banana and peanut butter smoothie with your choice of milk added 1 tsp of My GoldenrootTM (potassium, healthy fats, and protein)

Libido-Boosting Ingredients:

- Oysters (zinc)

- Dark chocolate (flavonoids and phenylethylamine)

- Strawberries (vitamin C and antioxidants)

- Avocado (healthy fats and potassium)

- Spinach (folate and iron)

- Garlic (allicin)

- Ginger (gingerol)

- Chili peppers (capsaicin)

- Omega-3 fatty acids

- My GoldenrootTM

- Vitamin C

- Vitamin E

- Folate

- Iron

- Zinc

- Potassium

- Complex carbohydrates

- Healthy fats

- Antioxidants

Remember, a balanced diet and healthy lifestyle are essential for balancing hormones and maintaining a healthy libido.

Hormone Imbalance Checklist:

Check off all that apply to get insight into your hormonal patterns

Estrogen Dominance

- Heavy, painful periods
- PMS symptoms (bloating, mood swings)
- Breast tenderness
- Weight gain around hips and thighs
- Fibroids, endometriosis

Low Estrogen

- Hot flashes, night sweats
- Vaginal dryness
- Low libido
- Fatigue
- Depression, mood swings

Low Progesterone

- Irregular menstrual cycles
- Insomnia
- Anxiety, irritability
- Spotting before periods
- Breast tenderness

High Testosterone

Acne

- Excess facial or body hair
- Scalp hair thinning
- Aggression or irritability
- Irregular menstrual cycles

Low Testosterone

- Fatigue, low energy
- Low libido
- Hair loss
- Muscle weakness
- Mood swings, depression
- Weight gain

High DHEA

- Oily skin, acne
- Excess hair growth in women
- Mood swings, irritability
- Aggressiveness
- Elevated libido

Low DHEA

- Low energy, chronic fatigue
- Poor stress response
- Low libido
- Weakened immune system
- Mood disturbances

High Cortisol

- Weight gain (especially abdominal)
- Insomnia, poor sleep
- Anxiety, irritability
- High blood pressure
- Sugar cravings

Low Cortisol

- Chronic fatigue
- Low blood pressure
- Dizziness, especially when standing
- Salt cravings
- Brain fog

Insulin Resistance

- Weight gain, especially around the belly
- Sugar cravings
- Fatigue after eating
- Dark patches of skin (acanthosis nigricans)
- High blood sugar
- Low Thyroid (Hypothyroidism)
- Fatigue, low energy
- Weight gain
- Cold intolerance
- Dry skin, thinning hair
- Depression, slow thinking

High Thyroid (Hyperthyroidism)

- Rapid heart rate
- Weight loss despite eating well
- Anxiety, restlessness
- Heat intolerance, sweating
- Tremors, insomnia

Low Vitamin D

- Fatigue, low energy
- Depression, mood swings
- Bone pain, muscle weakness
- Frequent infections
- Hair loss

Endocrine Disruptor Checklist

How many of these products do you use everyday? Consider switching to cleaner products that do not contain endocrine disruptors (List of common endocrine disruptors below).

Body Care Products

- Shampoos, conditioners
- Body washes, soaps

- Skin creams, lotions
- Deodorants, antiperspirants
- Sunscreens
- Perfumes, colognes
- Hair dyes, styling products
- Toothpaste

Make-up and Nail Care

- Foundation, concealer
- Lipsticks, lip balms
- Mascara, eyeliner, eyeshadow
- Nail polishes, removers
- Blush, bronzer, highlighter

Cleaning Products

- All-purpose cleaners
- Dish soaps
- Laundry detergents, fabric softeners
- Window cleaners
- Air fresheners, scented candles

Household Items

- Paints, varnishes
- Furniture (especially new or treated)
- Carpets, rugs (off-gassing chemicals)
- Non-stick cookware
- Plastic containers, wraps
- Toys (especially soft plastics)
- New electronics (off-gassing)
- Canned foods (BPA lining)
- Grocery receipts (thermal paper with BPA)

Food (High Pesticide Content)

- Strawberries, spinach, kale
- Peppers, grapes, cherries
- Apples, tomatoes, celery
- Peaches, pears, nectarines
- Bottled water (plastic leaching)

Job/Career

- Agricultural work (pesticides, herbicides)
- Landscaping, gardening

- Industrial cleaning
- Hairdressing (chemical treatments)
- Construction (paints, solvents)

Common Endocrine Disruptors:

Here's a list of common endocrine disruptors and their names you should look out for in products:

Common Endocrine Disruptors:

1. Parabens (Methylparaben, Ethylparaben, Propylparaben, Butylparaben)
2. Phthalates (DBP, DEP, DEHP, BBP, DiBP)
3. Bisphenols (BPA, BPS, BPF)
4. Triclosan and Triclocarban
5. PFAS (Perfluoroalkyl substances, often labeled as "stain-resistant" or "waterproof")
6. Formaldehyde and formaldehyde-releasing agents (DMDM Hydantoin, Quaternium-15)
7. Fragrance (Can contain multiple hidden chemicals, including phthalates)
8. Synthetic Musks (Galaxolide, Tonalide)
9. Brominated Flame Retardants (PBDEs)
10. Nonylphenols and Octylphenols

11. Perchlorate (found in packaging)

12. Pesticides (DDT, Atrazine, Glyphosate)

13. Dioxins (by-products from manufacturing and bleaching processes)

14. Polychlorinated Biphenyls (PCBs)

15. Heavy Metals (Lead, Mercury, Cadmium, Arsenic)

Checking product labels and opting for certified non-toxic, organic, or endocrine disruptor-free products can help reduce exposure to these harmful chemicals.

Access Our Hormone Testing

Saliva Testing

We offer comprehensive saliva hormone testing with an optional add on of a full thyroid panel. If your doctor will not test your hormones or you cannot access a full thyroid panel testing we can help. Our test is done in the comfort of your own home—no lab needed.

Saliva testing is the best way to accurately measure available hormones in the body.

www.soshormonehelp.com

Access Our Hormone Balancing Supplement Protocols

Follow the link to access our hormone balancing protocols for ease of selection and best pricing.

Access articles, checklists and additional resources for hormone balancing, digestive health and weight loss.

You can also choose to purchase your favorite brands of supplements for your whole family. They will be conveniently shipped to your door.

https://ca.fullscript.com/welcome/kathyryanrhn

To Purchase Goldenroot ™ please follow the link here.

https://manoticknaturalmarket.com/products/golden-root

MEET KATHY AND DARPAN

Darpan Ahluwalia is an award-winning Registered Holistic Nutritionist since 2002, Certified Live Blood Analyst, Functional Medicine Practitioner, and Herbalist specializing in gut and hormone health. She's been the owner/ operator of Manotick Natural Market since 2000 . She is the creator/ formulator of "My Goldenroot™, a unique turmeric blend supporting gut, liver, immune and brain health. Darpan has been honored as "Nutritionist of the Year" multiple times through Faces magazine and was named one of Canada's Top 50 Women by Distinctive Women of Canada. A mother of three and a fur baby, is also the Co-author of ContextEatingMethodTM weightloss. She offers counseling and education worldwide, empowering others through her extensive teaching, writing, and speaking engagements.

Kathy Ryan is a Registered Holistic Nutritionist since 2009 and the creator of the Context Eating Method, which provides women with a healthy and sustainable alternative to dieting. Over the course of her career she has worked with and been mentored by renowned health experts such as Dr. Maggie Yu and Lorna Vanderhaeghe.

Kathy speaks regularly at events, retreats, and corporate trainings. She spends her days helping clients worldwide to reverse chronic conditions and optimize hormone health. Living in rural Ontario, Kathy enjoys gardening, foraging, and spending time with her daughter, grandson and her dog Tesla.

Together, Darpan and Kathy are dedicated to guiding women on their wellness journeys using holistic approaches to balance hormones, nutrition, and lifestyle.

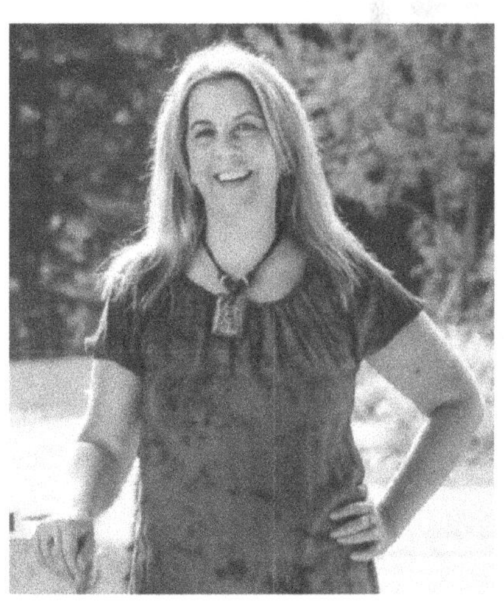

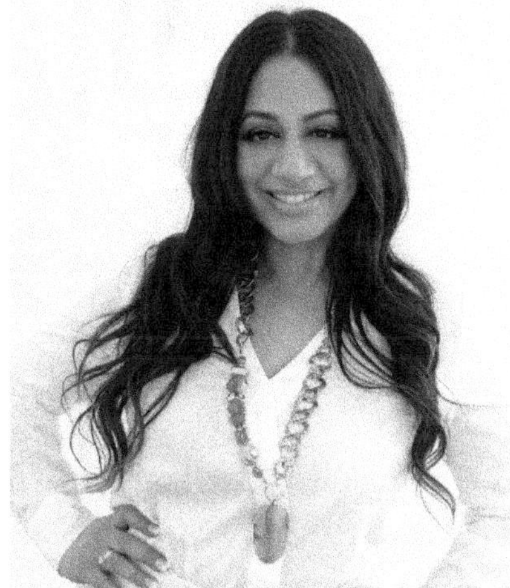

INVITE ME TO SPEAK: SOS FOR YOUR HORMONAL HOT MESS

If you would like me to speak to your audience about SOS for Your Hormonal Hot Mess, please reach out

HormoneBook.com

Instagram: @soshormonehelp
Website: HormoneBook.com
Email: contact@nutritionallynourished.com
More links: contexteatingmethod.com

thank you

Thank you for reading our book!

Dear Reader,

Well, you made it to the end—congrats! I hope you found some insights, a few laughs, and some practical steps that you can begin to implement to support your hormones and improve your overall health and wellbeing.

Sharing these strategies and insights to you, our clients, friends and beyond is a dream come true as it is our desire to positively impact tens of thousands of women worldwide.

Now, we need your help!

If you found value in these pages please take a minute to leave a 5-star review on Amazon. Not only will it make my day, but it'll also help this book get our message out to the world. Think of it as a little ripple effect—your review could be the exact thing someone needed to hear to pick up this book and read its life changing information.

Thanks so much for your support

Kathy and Darpan

MY GIFT TO YOU

I am so glad you're here!

As my Gift to you, get FREE Access to the Audiobook of SOS for Your Hormonal Hot Mess by scanning the QR Code below or visiting

HormoneBook.com/book